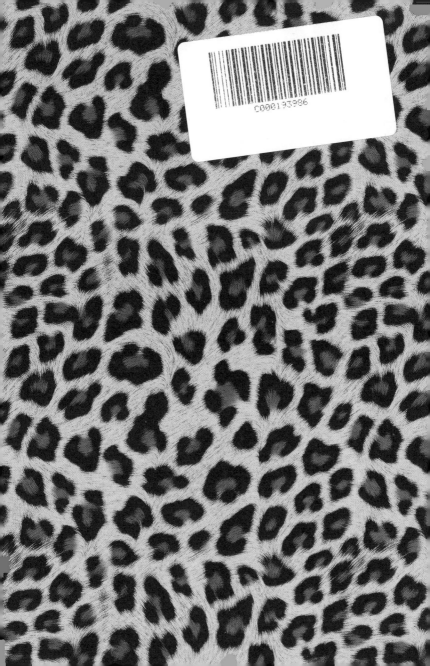

C000193986

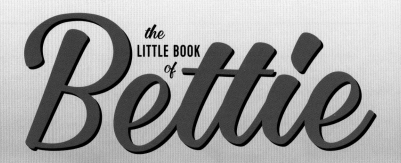

*the*
**LITTLE BOOK**
*of*
*Bettie*

**TAKING A** *Page* **FROM
THE QUEEN OF** **PINUPS**

*by*
**TORI RODRIGUEZ**

*foreword by*
**DITA VON TEESE**

**RUNNING PRESS**
PHILADELPHIA

Copyright © 2018 by Tori Rodriguez

Hachette Book Group supports the right to free expression and the value of copyright. The purpose of copyright is to encourage writers and artists to produce the creative works that enrich our culture.

The scanning, uploading, and distribution of this book without permission is a theft of the author's intellectual property. If you would like permission to use material from the book (other than for review purposes), please contact permissions@hbgusa.com. Thank you for your support of the author's rights.

Running Press
Hachette Book Group
1290 Avenue of the Americas, New York, NY 10104
www.runningpress.com
@Running_Press

Printed in China

First Edition: May 2018

Published by Running Press, an imprint of Perseus Books, LLC, a subsidiary of Hachette Book Group, Inc. The Running Press name and logo is a trademark of the Hachette Book Group.

The Hachette Speakers Bureau provides a wide range of authors for speaking events. To find out more, go to www.hachettespeakersbureau.com or call (866) 376-6591.

The publisher is not responsible for websites (or their content) that are not owned by the publisher.

Print book cover and interior design by Susan Van Horn.

Library of Congress Control Number: 2017957630

ISBNs: 978-0-7624-9151-3 (paperback), 978-0-7624-9150-6 (ebook)

1010

10  9  8  7  6  5  4  3  2  1

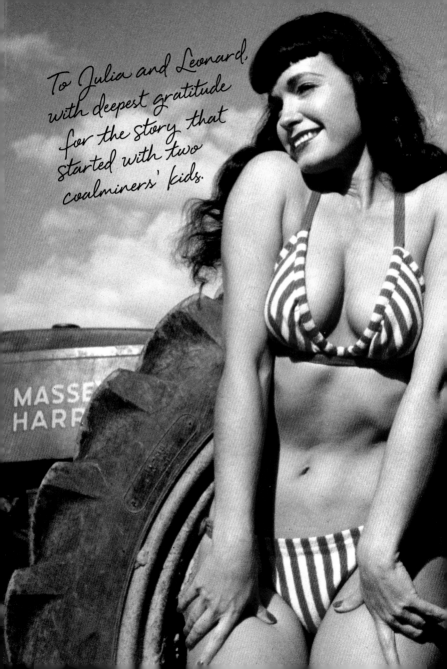

To Julia and Leonard,
with deepest gratitude
for the story that
started with two
coalminers' kids.

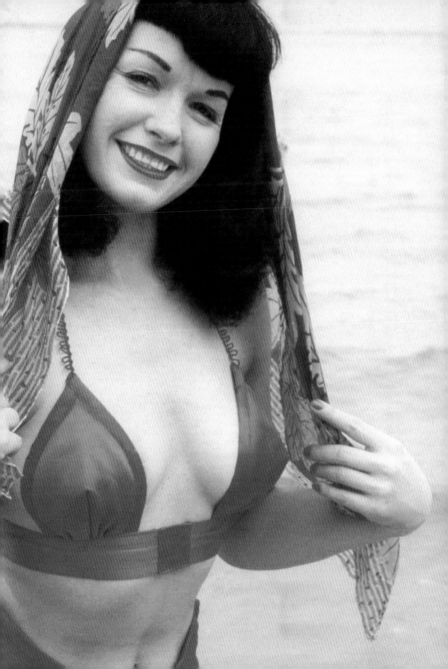

# CONTENTS

# FOREWORD
## by DITA VON TEESE

*B*ETTIE PAGE SPARKED MY TRANSFORMATION from Heather Sweet into Dita Von Teese in more ways than meet the eye. Bettie was her own woman. She was athletic. She had imperfect teeth and a slightly droopy eye. She was deemed short and too hippy to be a fashion model, by no less than Eileen Ford herself, who rejected Bettie for her agency. But despite not fitting within mainstream beauty standards, and despite the hard knocks of her childhood, Bettie Page lived on her own terms.

I first spotted her in a fetish magazine around 1990. I was captivated. Here was a woman genuinely smiling her way through pretty intense bondage scenes, and doing so with a mischief wrapped in warmth and humor. She was unabashed about her sexuality. For her shoots, she did her own makeup and hair and made her own bikinis and other costumes. That Bettie could do all of this while pushing the boundaries and having fun, and a lifetime later, have such a celebrated legacy, motivated me to at least give my own pipe dreams a try.

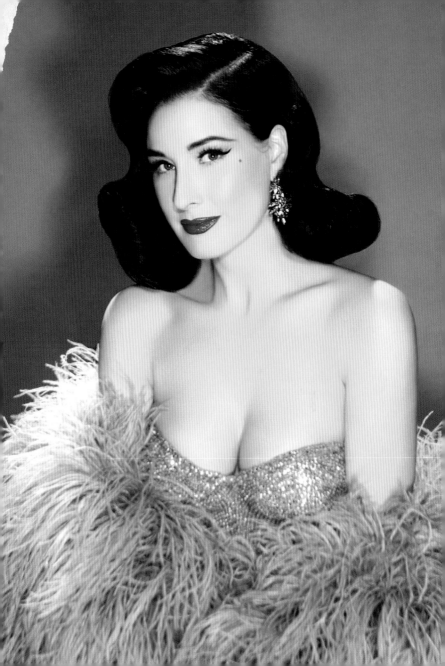

Launching my career as a modern-day incarnation of Bettie Page led to a radio show call with the actual woman herself. It remains among the great thrills of my life. Years later, Bettie invited me to go to church with her. Even during her modeling days, she attended church, as she didn't believe a God who put Adam and Eve here "as naked as jaybirds" would disapprove of nudity. I was living abroad, so I never did get to meet my muse, my hero.

Long before her kind invitation, I had let go of the literal homages to her. I'd realized, to truly honor Bettie Page meant going my own way. Bettie stood apart then and continues to do so now because she wasn't trying to be anyone but herself. If I was going to emulate anything about her, it would be how she lived: by her own convictions, exuding a strong will, coupled with a playful sensuality and generosity of spirit.

Some five years after Bettie died, I got a call about a suitcase under security in a Vegas warehouse that was part of the Irving Klaw Studios/Movie Stars News archives. It was filled with shoes from those infamous bondage shoots. It was also apparently headed for auction. I handwrote a letter to the owner explaining what it would mean for me to be the caretaker of a pair of her shoes. Faster than the crack of a whip, I was on a flight to look through the suitcase. Among the scruffy gems, they were there: those signature bump-toe black pumps with a distinct solid, sky-high heel that curved just so.

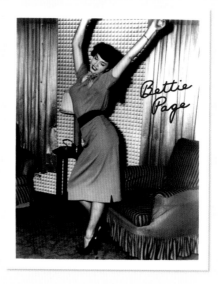

They are unlike anything I'd ever seen then or have seen since. Shoe size: six and a half. I wear size six and a half. These were the very same ones in those first snapshots of her I fell in love with. They came home with me that day. Did I try them on? Of course! But I don't wear them. They are a talisman, a lucky charm, the embodiment of how central Bettie Page remains in my life. (And no doubt in yours, since you're holding this book in your hands.) I occasionally share this treasure with guests at book signings or other appearances. After all, I'm not the only one who found myself because of Bettie Page.

*Dita Von Teese*

DECEMBER, 2017

I really
can't explain
it at all. I have
many fans—even
among teenagers, even
among young girls—
who claim I'm their
inspiration and
I've changed their
lives and everything.
It's very flattering
and uplifting and
I enjoy it.

—Bettie Page

# INTRODUCTION

*A*FTER A WILD-CHILD ADOLESCENCE, I must have decided at some point that I had better go ahead and hide that inner troublemaker away so I could have some semblance of a normal life, whatever that is. Along the path of college, grad school, marriage, divorce, motherhood, and career pursuits, that part of myself got further and further buried until I no longer felt connected to my inner spark. That light reignited instantly when I discovered Bettie Page several years ago. That may seem dramatic, but such bold statements are not uncommon among women who have embraced Bettie as a muse. Though her original fan base was mostly men, the community of female Bettie lovers has grown rapidly over the years to the point where we likely outnumber the guys now.

Because I'm a psychotherapist and a journalist, people frequently expressed surprise—I'd say some even scoffed—at the idea that I have a serious interest in the likes of Bettie Page. Taking a cue from her bravery, I ignored their judgments and pursued my growing interest in the Queen of Pinups. I published articles about her in various online and print magazines, wrote and recorded a song about her, and after connecting with CMG Worldwide, the company that licenses the use of her image, I began managing Bettie's official social media pages, as well as the blog on bettiepage.com.

Not long after, I got a license through CMG and started a Bettie-inspired fitness company. Through Bettie Page Fitness, I produced the first-ever body-positive workout videos, each of which is based on multiple Bettie poses and helps viewers cultivate her sense of confidence, strength, and joy. (You'll get a taste of these later in the book.) Ultimately, all of this led me here, getting to pay tribute to my main muse and write a book for my fellow Bettie Babes, both current and to-be. So, my scoffers were wrong, and so were Bettie's.

We are sold a lie that we must choose sides: professional or passionate; sensual or serious; promiscuous or chaste. It turns out that none of that is true, and the reason I know that is because Bettie walked this earth in her full glory, despite enduring numerous, truly hellish experiences. No matter what people told her she couldn't or shouldn't do in an era when many women—and men, for that matter—never questioned those prescriptions, she forged ahead with her heart as her trusty guide, and accidentally made history as a pioneer of empowerment, sexuality, and body positivity.

Bettie is the mirror that instantly reflects our potential back to us when we look at her. Once you get to know Bettie, you know that limitations are illusions and that hope can survive even the greatest hardships. One of the things I find most remarkable about Bettie's influence is that even though her fans idolize and adore her, she mostly inspires women not to be just like her but to be our authentic selves because that's the example she set. She lets us know that we really can have faith that if we stay true to who we are, it will all work out in the end.

Bettie spent her life just being herself—that seemingly basic thing that can actually be quite difficult. She embodied a simple complexity that often seemed contradictory. And isn't that the very point—to ultimately be that combination of things that makes you uniquely, gloriously you? That's why it's probably best that we can never quite nail down exactly what it is that makes Bettie a legend, because if we could, we would no doubt be tempted to copy it at the expense of what makes us unique, as Bettie was.

But that doesn't mean we can't take a page—or several—from her book by looking to her for inspiration in all areas of our lives. Let's explore the wonderful world of Bettie!

# *the*
# BETTIE
# BABES

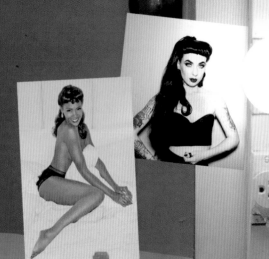

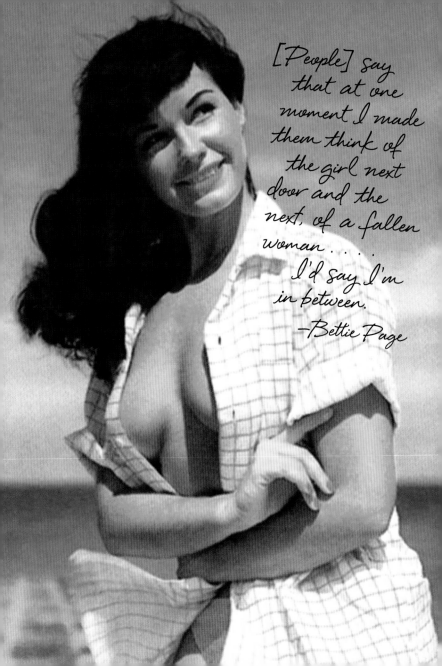

[People] say that at one moment I made them think of the girl next door and the next, of a fallen woman . . . . I'd say I'm in between.
—Bettie Page

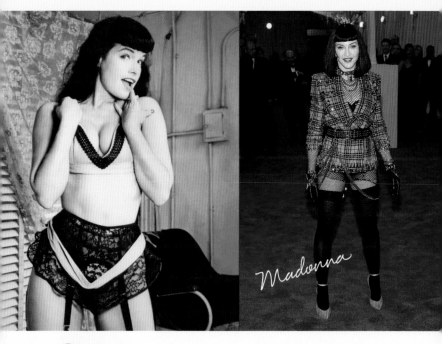

Madonna

*W*HAT IS IT ABOUT BETTIE?" is an all-too-common question that just about anyone who knows about her will ultimately ponder. The answer is both obvious and elusive at the same time. There are a million reasons to admire her, but it's impossible to pinpoint the precise thing that fuels her fans' intense allegiance. "When I first saw photos of Bettie Page when I was a teenager, she had such a magical quality that drew me to her. I saw a beautiful, radiant, and confident woman, and the more I learned about her the more she

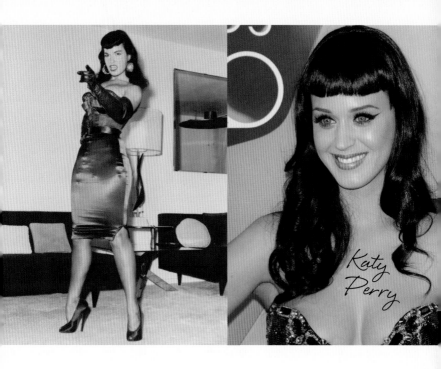

Katy Perry

inspired me," said Miss Lady Lace, a pinup model, burlesque artist, and vintage blogger in Perth, Australia. "She has a special element that's difficult to put into words."

Think about this: Is there any other person in history who has scores of devotees worldwide walking around looking just like them? And that includes several top icons of the current era. Katy Perry sported a straight-up Bettie look for a long stretch of her career, and Madonna has rocked the hair and other Bettie-inspired touches (fishnets-and-

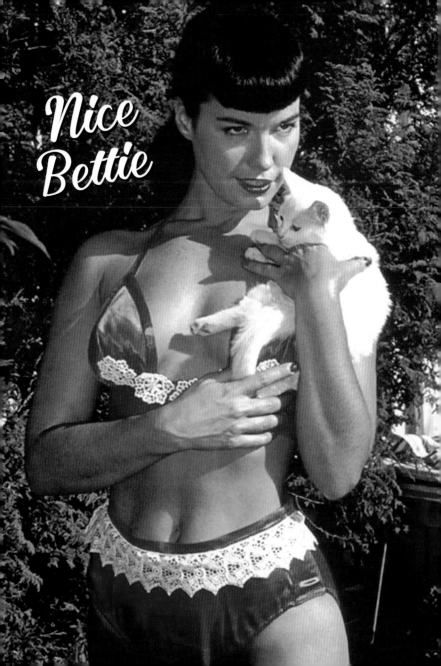

gloves combo, the cone bra, fetish boots) numerous times. In 2014, these two stars even teamed up for a Bettie-inspired photo shoot for *V* magazine.

> "When I put on the Bettie Page wig, I got into the character. I started researching Bettie Page and tried to channel her pinups and poses."
>
> —*Beyoncé*

Beyoncé has donned a full-on Bettie persona in three different music videos, first for the song "Video Phone" from her album *I Am . . . Sasha Fierce*, then again as a guest star in Lady Gaga's video for "Telephone." In a 2010 *W* magazine article in which she talks about the "seven looks that shaped her career," her homages to Bettie make the list twice. She told the interviewer, "When I put on the Bettie Page wig, I got into the character. I started researching Bettie Page and tried to channel her pinups and poses."

Queen Bey took it even further in her video for "Why Don't You Love Me," replicating the Queen of Pinups's appearance and performance from a 1950s stag film produced by Irving Klaw. She recalled: "I was still thinking about Bettie Page, and wanted to do something that was inspired by her. This video was a secret: I paid for and

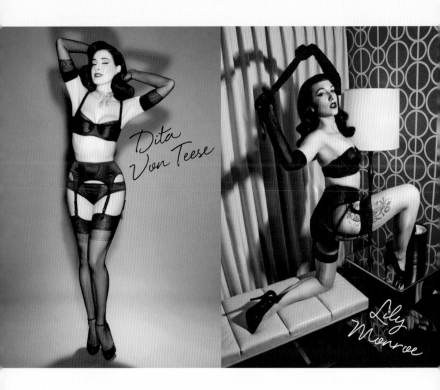

*Dita Von Teese*

*Lily Monroe*

codirected it and didn't tell my label or my management. The clothes and jewelry are from my closet, the wigs are mine, and I did my own makeup."

International burlesque sensation Dita Von Teese began her career as a Bettie look-alike before evolving into her own unique style. "Bettie Page was my very first inspiration. When I first saw her picture in a fetish shop in 1990, the first thing I noticed was her distinctive style," she told me. "But what really fascinated me and kept my attention was much

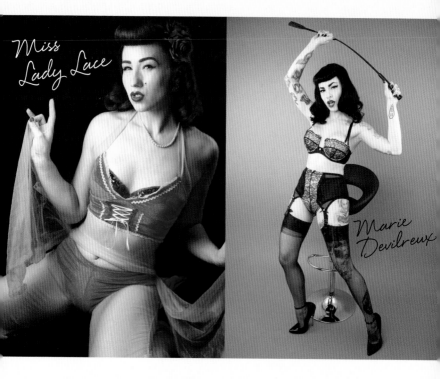

*Miss Lady Lace*

*Marie Devilreux*

more than that. It was her sense of playfulness, her warmth and humor in those intense bondage and fetish scenes that really made me understand what captivates a viewer."

Most likely it's the combination of traits, including ones that seem conflicting, that contribute to that inexplicable Bettie magic. According to women who love Bettie, a huge part of her appeal is, in fact, this very ability to embody what we view as opposing qualities, to pull off something we are constantly told can't be done.

"And here was this woman who had dark hair, curves, and people loved her. It was at that exact moment that I started to give up all of those old, impossible ideals I had set for myself and began to accept myself as I was."

—*BrittanyJean*

To many of these gals, their love of Bettie extends beyond simple admiration or even fangirl adoration. They will tell you she has literally changed their lives— even helped them recover from their own struggles and deep-seated societal conditioning. When someone told a glammed-up BrittanyJean, a pinup model from North Carolina who runs a blog called *Perfectly Pinned Up*, that she looked like Bettie Page during a night out, she looked her up when she got home. "I was stunned! She wasn't the initial idea of what I thought beauty was at the time. I had grown up wanting to model, I starved myself to keep my weight down, and thought I would never be beautiful because it seemed all the women considered beautiful were blonde, tan, and super thin," she recalls. "And here was this woman who had dark hair, curves, and people loved her. It was at that exact moment that I started to give

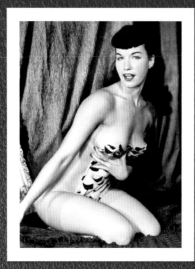

# JUST ENOUGH TO COVER UP

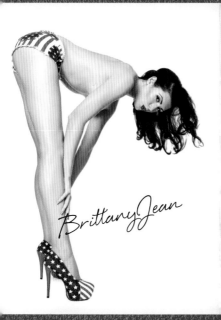

Brittany Jean

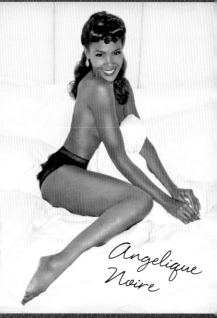

Angelique Noire

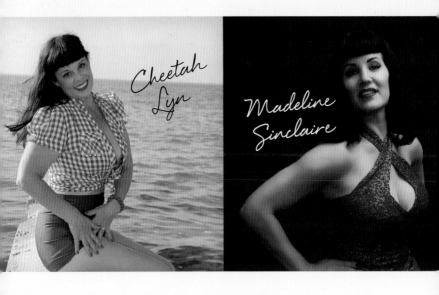

*Cheetah Lyn*

*Madeline Sinclaire*

up all of those old, impossible ideals I had set for myself and began to accept myself as I was."

"Her down-to-earth vibe mixed with the naughty but girlish vibe, captivated me . . ."

— *Angelique Noire*

How liberating to have an instant, explicit reminder that women have far more choices than we presumed, that we are not nearly as limited in what we can express or achieve as we were made to believe—that we don't have to choose one or the other, after all. It was this surprising blend of traits that

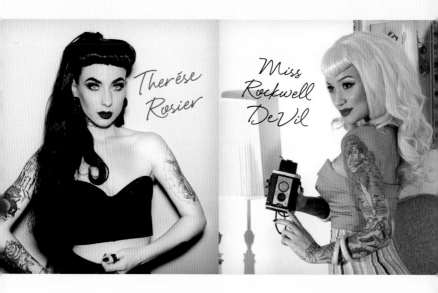

Thérése Rosier

Miss Rockwell DeVil

drew in Angelique Noire, a LA-based model. "Her down-to-earth vibe mixed with the naughty but girlish vibe, captivated me," she explains. "She always seemed in control, even while tied up. She seemed to know how to communicate so many different feelings without saying a word."

We have been told we can't or shouldn't be this and that at the same time, and yet there was Bettie—back in the even more sexist and stifling 1950s, mind you—plainly and rightfully calling bullshit on that notion simply by looking how she did and being exactly who she was. "I loved the way her attitude could easily shift from dominant to submissive, with each role an underlying sense of humor and amusement with herself," says Von Teese. "Yes, she was beautiful,

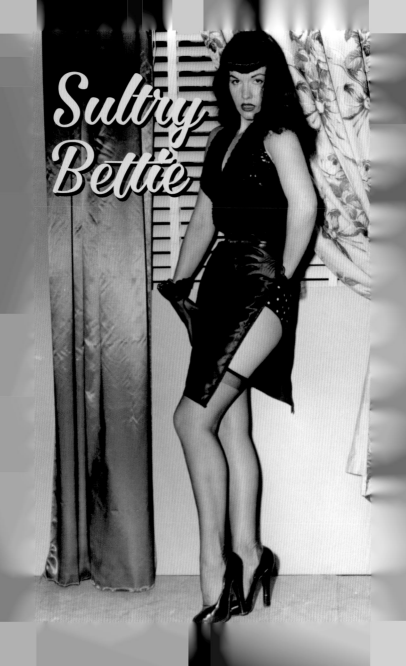

*Sultry Bettie*

but there are so many more reasons that she's managed to inspire generation after generation."

It can be tremendously liberating to claim such a vast range of expression and emotion against the backdrop of restrictive gender expectations. It tells us there's much more to explore beneath the surface—in both Bettie and ourselves. I doubt many women have learned about Bettie without also learning a lot about themselves.

"Learning more about her life and the way she tackled obstacles cheerfully—and without a care in the world about

> "Learning more about her life and the way she tackled obstacles cheerfully—and without a care in the world about what others thought—has inspired me to have an optimistic attitude ..."
> — *Sunny Moon*

what others thought—has inspired me to have an optimistic attitude and, more importantly, to take everyone's opinion with a grain of salt," shares Young Sun Moon, an acupuncturist, yoga teacher, makeup artist, and model who also goes by the pinup name Sunny Moon. "Nobody will ever be happy all the time, but it is the attitude with which you face circumstances that makes the difference in how you feel about an outcome."

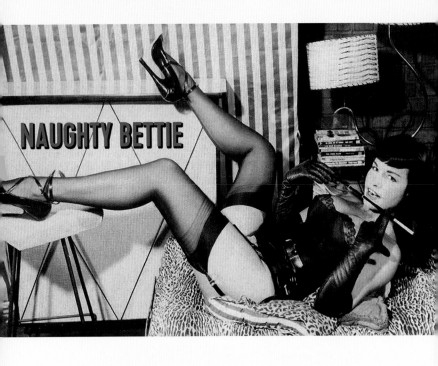

# NAUGHTY BETTIE

For Boston-based model Jenny Mostly, Bettie made all the difference in her self-concept after she discovered her in junior high school. She recalls that when she was a young girl, Barbie was the ideal—thin, blonde, and with a permanent smile. Bettie showed her a more realistic alternative: "A real woman isn't always smiling—it's okay for her to be playful or pouty and relay her personality and emotions," she realized. Learning about Bettie led her to the understanding that "Beauty is not a single ideal, but rather something uncovered by confidence and inner

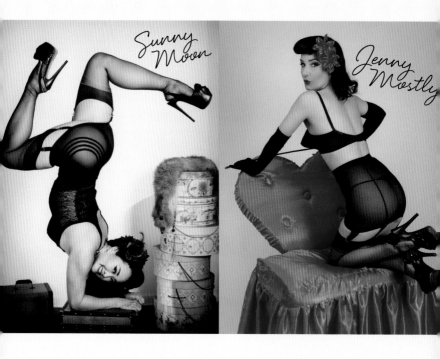

*Sunny Moon*

*Jenny Mostly*

strength. She allowed me to explore my being with sincerity at a most crucial time."

This is a common theme among female Bettie fans: not only is she an inspiration but a clear example of how to be in the world, when women are faced with an infinite list of

"Beauty is not a single ideal, but rather something uncovered by confidence and inner strength."
— *Jenny Mostly*

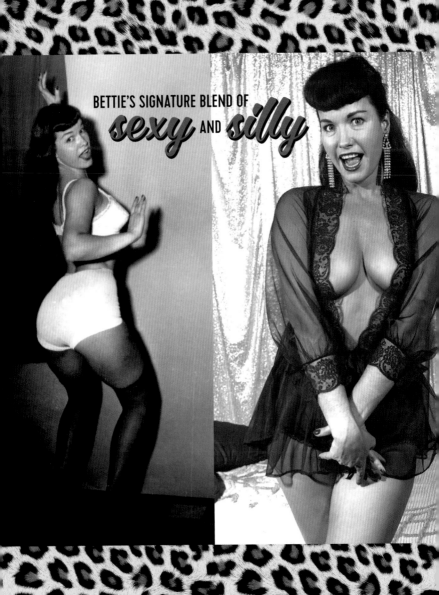

BETTIE'S SIGNATURE BLEND OF *sexy* AND *silly*

what not to do and how not to act, but with very few realistic or appealing counterexamples of womanhood. For some, Bettie has served as what philosophers and psychologists call an archetype. Fittingly, the literal meaning of this word is "the original pattern or model from which all things of the same kind are copied or on which they are based; a model or first form; prototype."

Today, women show their Bettie love in lots of different ways, including incorporating elements of her appearance, often with their own twist. While plenty of women rock a classic Bettie look—the black hair and U-shaped bangs and traditional, simple makeup and outfits, other gals mash it up with tattoos (including ones of the pinup queen herself!), piercings, edgier makeup like exaggerated brows, and more dramatic hair—like a Bettie 'do but in bright blue or pink. Then there are lots of pinups who have a Bettie look in their repertoire, which they alternate or combine with other popular pinup styles, like victory rolls or a front wave.

Not only are women adopting aspects of her appearance; we are also channeling her joyfulness and lightheartedness, right along with her strength, resilience, and bravery to help guide our careers, relationships, and even recovery from emotional and physical issues.

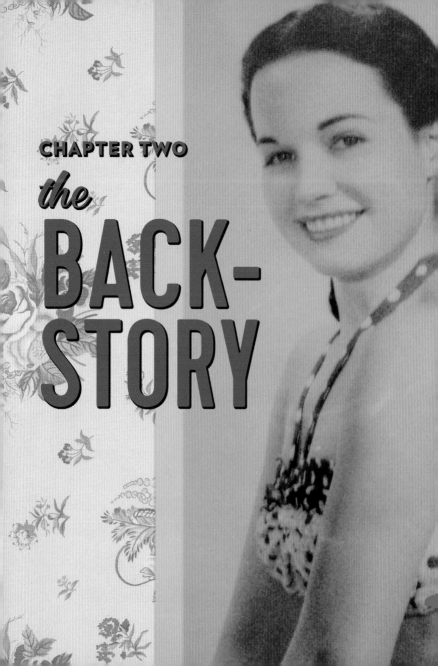

CHAPTER TWO

*the*

# BACK-
# STORY

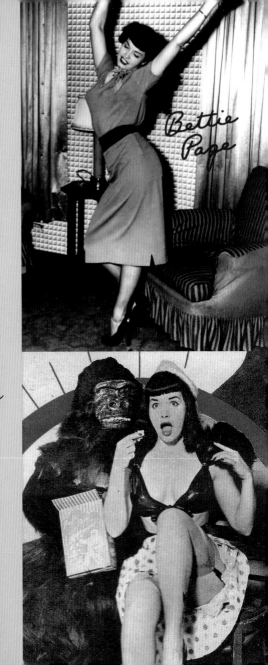

I think you can do your own thing as long as you're not hurting anybody else—that's been my philosophy ever since I was a little girl.

—Bettie Page

Bettie Page

*I*T'S HARD TO BELIEVE that a woman with such far-reaching influence on modern culture was born nearly a century ago. Bettie Mae Page entered this world on April 22, 1923, in Nashville, Tennessee, and her journey from there to international pinup fame was marked by intense struggle. She was the second of the six Page children, and her family was so poor they often went without food.

Money got even tighter for the family when her parents divorced. When Bettie was ten, she and her two sisters, Gloria and Joyce (nicknamed Goldie and Lub), were sent to live in an orphanage for about a year until their mother, Edna, could afford to support them again. This may be the first glimpse of Bettie's tendency to turn lemons into lemonade: While at the orphanage, she and her sisters made up a game called "Program," in which they would imitate celebrity poses they saw in the newspaper. "I guess that's where I started learning how

PREVIOUS SPREAD, BACKGROUND: An early modeling photo of pre-bangs Bettie in 1949; courtesy Mark Mori, *Bettie Page Reveals All;* UPPER RIGHT: Dancing Bettie; LOWER RIGHT: Cropping from a 1950's "girlie mag."

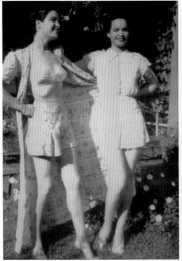 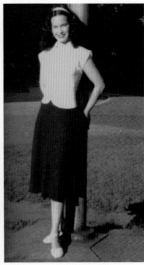

FROM LEFT: Bettie and her sister Goldie practicing modeling poses as teenagers • Bettie as a young woman, not long before she forever altered *hairstory* by adopting her signature bangs

to pose," Bettie recalled in a 1996 interview. "I just always knew what to do with my body."

The girls finally reunited with their mother but still faced ongoing hunger and hardship. For extra income, Edna allowed Bettie's father, Roy, to rent a room in their house. Despite any financial savings that may have come from this arrangement, Bettie and her sisters paid a steep price: she revealed in her later years that Roy began molesting her when she was thirteen, and that he had abused the other girls in the same way.

Bettie found a safe place in her local community center, where her now-famous DIY approach was no doubt fortified. This is where she learned how to sew, a skill that would come in handy years later when she created her own homemade bikinis and lingerie. (She once said she didn't like how the store-bought stuff fit her, so she preferred to make her own.) She also spent lots of time there reading and doing homework.

Somehow, even with a growling belly and traumatic home life, Bettie managed to excel academically at Hume-Fogg High School, a Nashville school for high achievers that still operates today. Besides maintaining a stellar GPA, she was involved in a range of school activities, serving as program director of the drama club and coeditor of the yearbook and student newspaper. Her ambition earned her the title of "Girl Most Likely to Succeed" in her junior and senior years.

Bettie's dedication to her studies almost snagged her the top spot of valedictorian, along with the full scholarship to Vanderbilt University that would have come with the title. Alas, after she skipped an art class to attend a rehearsal for a play, her class grade dropped to a B, bringing her GPA down to a maddening one-quarter below the average required of the valedictorian. She was crushed when the scholarship went to another student.

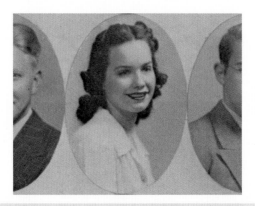

PAGE, BETTIE MAI
*"The secret of success is constancy of purpose."*
Academic-Commercial; Dramatic Club, '38, '39, '40, Production Manager,
'40; College Club, '39, '40, Program Chairman, '39, '40; Pep Club, '39;
Student Council, '37, '38, '39, Secretary and Treasurer, '39; Regimental
Sponsor of R. O. T. C., '39; Smartest Girl Sophomore, '38; Smartest Girl
and Girl Most Likely to Succeed in Junior Class, '39; Girl Most Likely
to Succeed in Senior Class, '40; D. A. R. Winner, '40; Co-Editor of Senior
*Echo*, '40; Salutatorian, '40; Girls' Declamatory Contest, '39, '40; Hume
Debate, '40; *Fogg Horn* Staff, '38, '39, '40, Co-Editor, '39, '40; President
of Session Room, '38, '39; Honor Roll, '37, '38, '39, '40

Bettie's high school yearbook photo, 1940: "Most Likely to Succeed"

Still, with the second-place salutatorian title, Bettie received a partial scholarship to Peabody College (now a part of Vanderbilt). Those funds covered the first year, then she worked her way through the other three as a secretary for a Civil War novelist before graduating with a bachelor's degree in 1944. During that era, less than 4 percent of women were college graduates. The year before she graduated, Bettie married her sweetie of two years, Billy Neal, not long before he was drafted into the navy amid World War II.

Right after receiving her diploma, Bettie moved to San Francisco where her new hubby was stationed. The way Bettie tells it, the marriage was plagued by jealous and controlling behavior from Billy, "whom I should never have married in the first place," she told a reporter. After asking the reporter if she planned to get married, she said she wasn't sure, so Bettie left her with some closing advice: "Well, don't be a fool and marry the first guy that asks you," she warned, laughing.

In 1947, Bettie divorced Billy and soon after moved to New York City, where she rented her own little apartment and supported herself with secretarial work while dreaming of becoming a movie star like her favorite actress, Bette Davis. A couple of years earlier, she had been invited to make a screen test at 20th Century Fox, but nothing came of it. She thought it might have had something to do with the way they did her hair and makeup—which she said was awful and made her resemble a caricature of Joan Crawford— instead of letting her do it herself. The Hollywood execs were reportedly not fond of Bettie's robust Southern accent, either. On top of all that, she had to spurn a sleazy producer's fame-for-favors proposition before it was all over.

Bettie continued to long for screen stardom, later taking on a theater apprenticeship and acting mostly in stage plays. Ultimately, the acting dream never fully materialized, and that was one of her only regrets in life. Bettie's other big disappointment was not having children. She said she always wanted to have three but couldn't because of what her doctor said was a hormone imbalance.

In her early days in New York, Bettie suffered yet another devastating trauma when she accepted a guy's invitation to go dancing—one of her very favorite pastimes—and ended up being trapped in a car with five men, who took her to an isolated area and sexually assaulted her. As she always had before, Bettie did the best she could to move on and continued plugging away at the secretarial grind until her modeling career took off quite unexpectedly.

"Bettie, you've got a very high forehead. I think you'd look good if you cut some bangs to cover it."

—*Jerry Tibbs*

Though she had done a bit of fashion modeling, her pinup stardom all began with a walk on the beach at Coney Island in 1950. She noticed a man working out and stopped to watch him do his thing for a while. He turned out to be Jerry Tibbs, an African American police officer who enjoyed photography as a hobby. They struck up a conversation, and he offered to get Bettie's pinup portfolio started by snapping some shots of her.

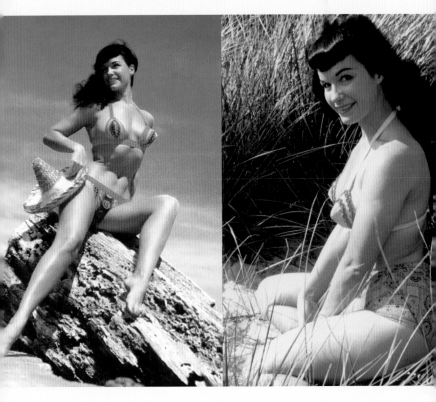

Tibbs soon suggested the essential image tweak that would make history. As Bettie recalled: "For years, I had my hair parted down the middle in a ponytail tucked down around the sides. But he said to me, 'Bettie, you've got a very high forehead. I think you'd look good if you cut some bangs to cover it.' Well, I went and cut the bangs, and I've been wearing them ever since. They say it's my trademark."

Tibbs introduced Bettie to other shutterbugs, and she

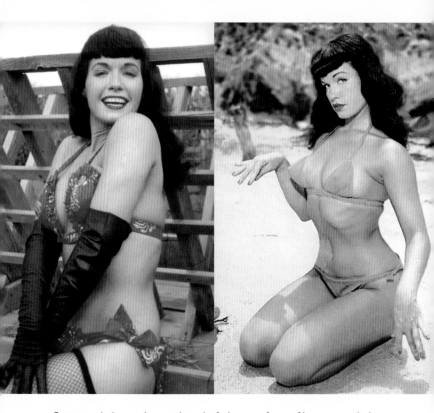

Bettie tended to snub store-bought fashions in favor of her own, including these pointy-boobed two-pieces (at a time when bikinis were considered highly risqué); a yellow two-piece; and a red bikini with opera gloves and fishnets. She would often mix such unexpected items like opera gloves and fishnets.

quickly became the fave of camera clubs (especially because she was uninhibited about nudity and more than happy to lose her threads upon request), girlie mags, and fetish photographer Irving Klaw. When she realized she could make a

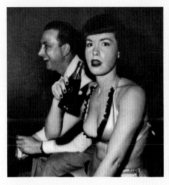 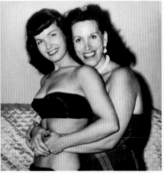

FROM LEFT: Rare candid with photographer Irving Klaw during a break on set. Bettie was fond of both Mr. Klaw and his sister Paula, who paid and treated her well. • With Paula Klaw, who Bettie said was one of the nicest women she'd ever met. OPPOSITE: Bettie's look ranged from angelic to dangerous, with lots of variation in between. Check out the cute toe rings in the photo at left on page 43.

lot more money in a fraction of the time by posing for camera clubs versus sitting at a desk for forty hours a week, she promptly ditched the secretarial job. This alone was a pretty radical mind-set for a woman in that era—she knew her own value, and she prioritized her free time so that she could travel to visit family and generally enjoy life.

She took a shot at mainstream modeling but was supposedly turned down by Eileen Ford for being too short and "hip-y." She worked regularly for Klaw and his sister, Paula, for several years, posing coyly in her DIY costumes most of the time. She also did her own hair and makeup when she modeled. In no time, Bettie became known as the "Queen of Pinups."

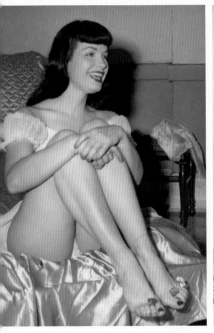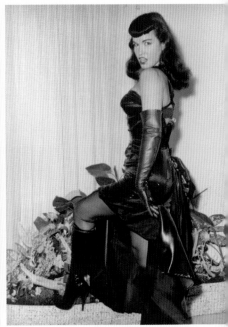

As part of her job requirements as a Klaw model, Bettie also posed in S&M-style fetish wear (think thigh-high boots with impossible heels, corsets, and patent leather) for bondage photos Klaw produced for private clients—including doctors and lawyers, as Bettie recalled. In these photos, she is sometimes the fierce and fearsome dominatrix, poised to spank a fellow model or posing with a mean face and whip in hand. Other times, she is submissive as the spankee or even trussed up with a ball gag in her mouth.

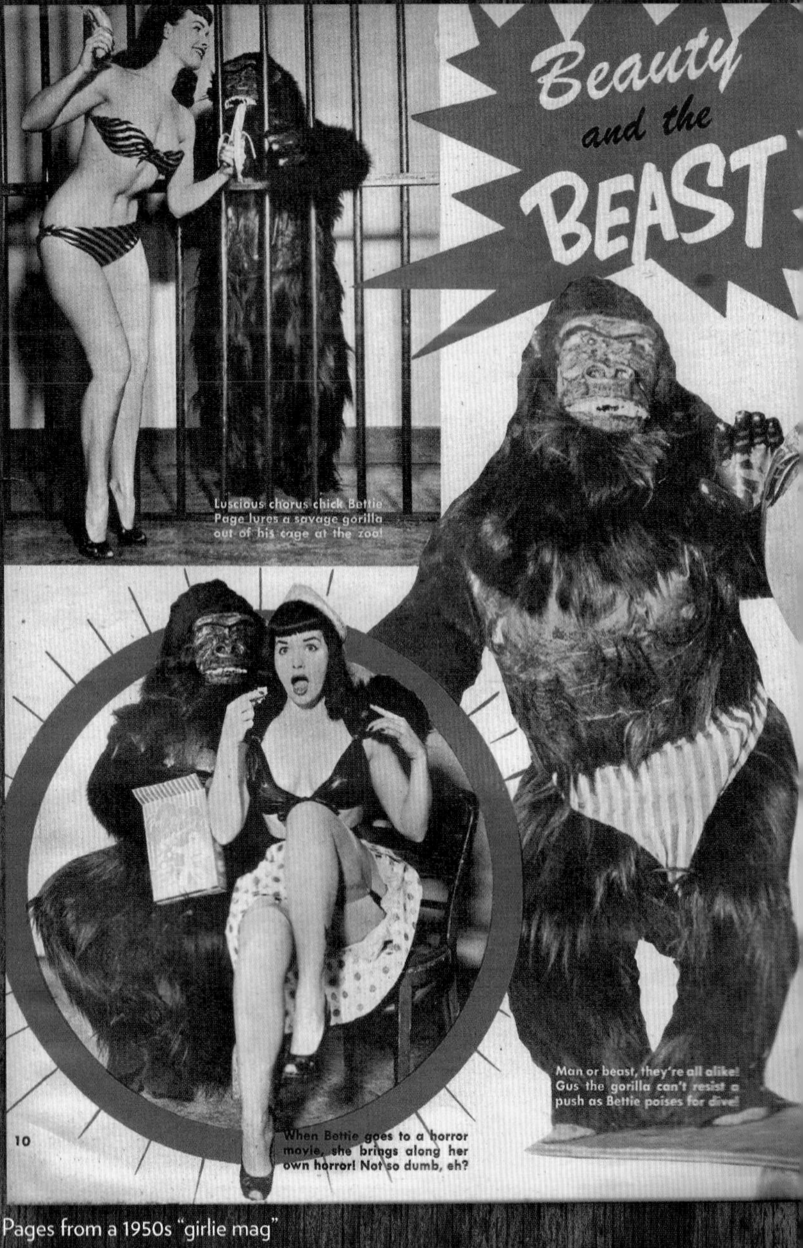

Beauty and the BEAST

Luscious chorus chick Bettie Page lures a savage gorilla out of his cage at the zoo!

When Bettie goes to a horror movie, she brings along her own horror! Not so dumb, eh?

Man or beast, they're all alike! Gus the gorilla can't resist a push as Bettie poises for dive!

10

Pages from a 1950s "girlie mag"

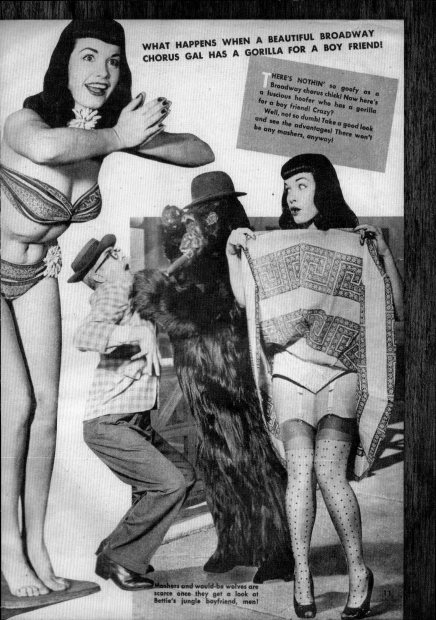

# WHAT HAPPENS WHEN A BEAUTIFUL BROADWAY CHORUS GAL HAS A GORILLA FOR A BOY FRIEND!

THERE'S NOTHIN' so goofy as a Broadway chorus chick! Now here's a luscious hoofer who has a gorilla for a boy friend! Crazy? Well, not so dumb! Take a good look and see the advantages! There won't be any mashers, anyway!

Mashers and would-be wolves are scarce once they get a look at Bettie's jungle boyfriend, men!

11

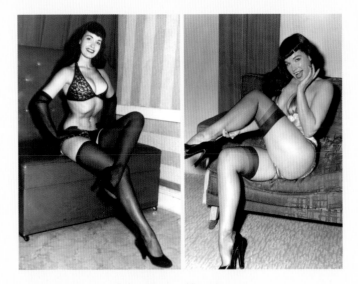

ABOVE AND OPPOSITE: Relatively tame Klaw photos

What many fans find remarkable—and is a major part of Bettie's unique appeal—is that in just about any role, she maintained her cheerful attitude and didn't seem to take any of it seriously. As Dita Von Teese told me when I interviewed her for an article I wrote for theatlantic.com: "You see her going back and forth between this fun-loving character to a stern dominatrix. . . . She had this ability to bring a playful quality to something that was very taboo (whether nudity or bondage), and you could tell she was in control—even hog-tied and ball-gagged, you sense she can get out whenever she wants."

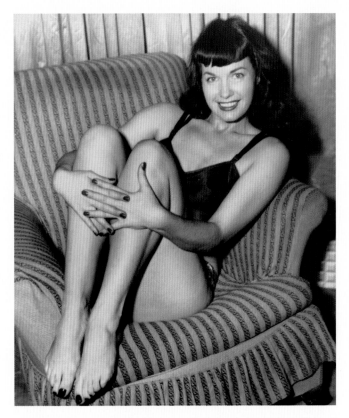

Government officials, however, did take the fetish photos seriously, and the Klaw gig came to a halt not long after Senator Estes Kefauver, a 1952 US presidential candidate, led what has been described as a witch hunt against sexual expression—or "indecency," as he called it—in hopes of winning support from voters. Klaw's work was considered pornographic at

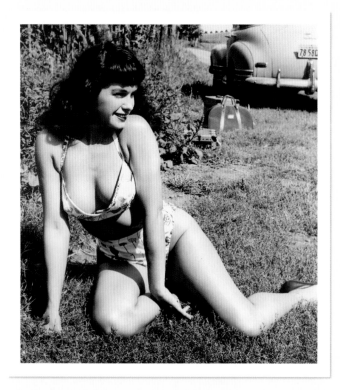

THIS SPREAD: Photographed by notorious NYC photographer Weegee

that time, even when no lady bits were visible, and he became a prime target for Kefauver. The feds ultimately did not prosecute Klaw, but the prolonged ordeal destroyed his business and, according to Bettie, his health and his life.

Bettie was subpoenaed to testify before a Senate committee as a part of the investigation but was not called at the

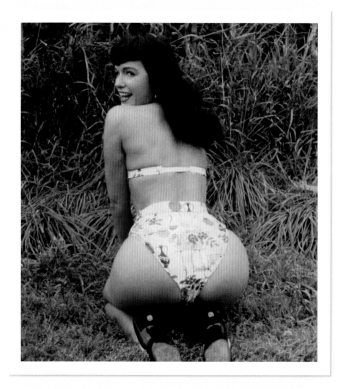

hearing, and she never got in trouble for any of the Klaw photos. But she was plenty distraught and disgusted at the unfair treatment of her boss and the implication that she was doing something immoral. Fortunately, the experience did little to dampen her career, though it was believed to be a contributing factor in her eventual decision to quit modeling. In hindsight, she has been lauded as a key figure

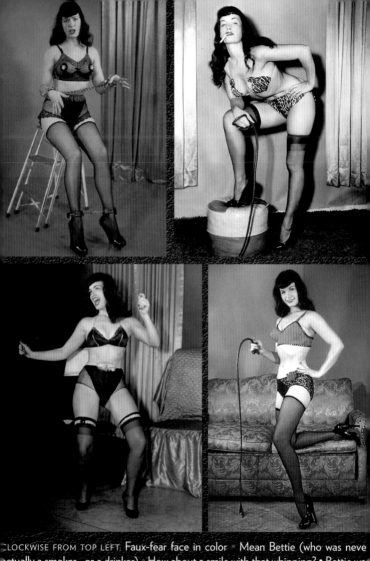

CLOCKWISE FROM TOP LEFT: Faux-fear face in color • Mean Bettie (who was neve
actually a smoker—or a drinker) • How about a smile with that whipping? • Bettie was
a dancing queen and loved ballroom styles, among other types.

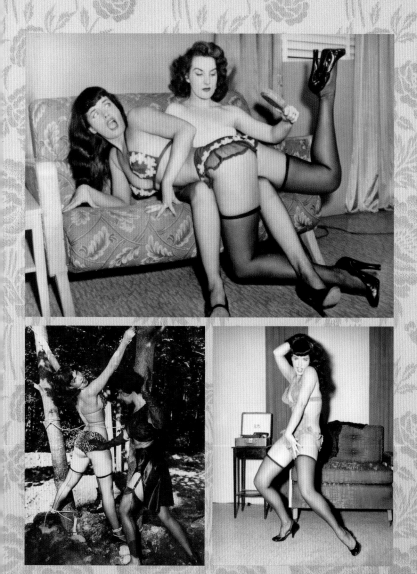

CLOCKWISE FROM TOP LEFT: Bettie's faux-fear face • More of that Bettie boogie • Bondage Bettie giving a look that says, "Seriously?!" Those Klaw clients meant business about that rope play, it seems.

THE LITTLE BOOK OF BETTIE

in opening the door to the sexual revolution of the 1960s, thanks to her rare, free-spirit approach to nudity and sexuality that contrasted so sharply with all norms of her era.

Over time, Bettie had begun working with other renowned photographers, including the actor, comedian, and producer Harold Lloyd, and the crime photographer known as Weegee. Bettie also made a legendary connection with Florida-based Bunny Yeager, previously a pinup model herself who discovered that she had more of a passion for looking through the lens than at it. Bettie's work with Bunny—especially the jungle-themed photos and those shot at the beach and an amusement park—is now perhaps her most widely celebrated and most appreciated by mainstream audiences.

## By 1957, Bettie had gotten her fill of the modeling life, later saying she felt there were just *too* many photos of her.

Perhaps the most well-known shot of Bettie by Bunny is the Christmas photo that shows Bettie in her birthday suit, rocking a Santa hat and winking at the camera as she hangs an ornament on a Christmas tree. Bunny submitted it to *Playboy*, and it became the centerfold of the January 1955 issue, just a little over a year after Hugh Hefner launched his risqué magazine. Hef, as he was casually known, would turn out to be a valuable connection for Bettie later in life.

By 1957, Bettie had gotten her fill of the modeling life, later saying she felt there were just *too* many photos of her. (She has been cited as the most photographed model in history.) Plus, she wanted to give teaching a go since that's what she went to college for, but it didn't take her long to realize that wasn't her thing.

Though she was in greater demand than ever, Bettie left the pinup life behind and moved to Florida, where she married Armon Walterson—a guy twelve years her junior— in 1958. She hadn't dated much during her modeling days and may have been overeager to settle down. However, she eventually realized she and Armon had little in common; he reportedly only cared about hamburgers and sex, the latter of which she said she taught him all about. The gulf between them grew even wider when Bettie became a born-again Christian on New Year's Eve, 1959. Armon wanted no part of this, and the couple divorced in 1963.

That same year, back in her hometown of Nashville, Bettie remarried Billy Neal, very briefly, before the marriage was again dissolved. Bettie found a deep sense of gratitude and purpose in religious studies, and at various points she attended Bible college, taught Bible school, and worked or volunteered for the famed evangelist Billy Graham. She had hoped to be a missionary but she was rejected for having been divorced. She thought it might help if she remarried Billy, but it didn't pan out that way.

Bettie returned to Peabody to earn a master's degree in English, but when she was just a few credits shy of graduating, she became too overwhelmed juggling her studies and abandoned that goal. She decided to move back to Florida, where she met Harry Lear while out dancing one night. He became her third husband in 1967. From Bettie's descriptions in various interviews, Harry was the closest she came to a true love, but their marriage was fraught with problems, first because of his ex-wife's relentless, jealousy-fueled harassment of Bettie. Lear's lack of intervention in the sticky situation led Bettie to lose respect for him.

Bettie also began to experience severe mental health issues while living with Harry and his three children from his first marriage, and she was diagnosed with paranoid schizophrenia. In one situation described in the posthumous documentary that she narrated, *Bettie Page Reveals All*, she threatened the family with a knife while having religious-themed hallucinations. That led to her confinement in a Florida psychiatric ward for six months.

Bettie and Harry divorced in 1972, but even after the split, Harry continued to take care of her and allowed her to stay in the house until she was able to find a place to live. For many years afterward, Bettie faced poverty and additional stints in psychiatric hospitals. Most notably, she spent nearly ten years at Patton State Hospital in California after being found not guilty by reason of insanity for an incident in which she attacked a landlord with a knife during a psychotic episode.

# Bettie lived in obscurity until a resurgence in her fame picked up in the 1980s and '90s.

She tried to keep these problems secret for many years, but she spoke about the experience in her documentary, recalling how terrible the antipsychotic drugs made her feel and how she was ashamed to talk about it for so long. "It wasn't like it is today," she said in the film, alluding to the stigma of society's perception of mental illness, which while still an issue today, was even worse in Bettie's time.

After many years of struggle, Bettie finally stabilized and was able to live a low-key life. She lived in obscurity until a resurgence in her fame picked up in the 1980s and '90s. Often credited as the key factor in this rediscovery is the Bettie-based character (named Betty) by artist Dave Stevens in his comic *The Rocketeer*, which became a Disney movie in 1991. Stevens became one of her closest friends, and they spent a fair amount of time together before his death from leukemia only months before Bettie's passing in 2008.

That newfangled invention now known as the Internet was also emerging around the time of the renewed focus on Bettie, and people were sharing her photos in large numbers. Her influence was making its way into fashion shows, movies, and celeb photo shoots. Loads of products bearing her name and image were popping up everywhere, but Bettie wasn't seeing a cent of the profits until that early ally Hugh Hefner put her in touch with an entertainment attorney friend of his. Mark Roesler is the founder of CMG Worldwide, a company that specializes in licensing images of a long list of deceased celebrities, including Jayne Mansfield, James Dean, Josephine Baker, Ingrid Bergman, and Bette Davis (Bettie's idol!). He became Bettie's friend and agent, and still represents her estate to this day.

> ## "She had the courage to do something no one else was doing."
> —*Johnny Rotten*

With Roesler's help, Bettie finally had financial stability in later life and was able to bask in several years of adoration from fans, whom she enjoyed interacting with in letters and on public chat room–style interviews. She liked to stay up late at night watching old movies—especially Westerns and other Hollywood classics. Even in her older age, she would create fitness routines to do at home, and she read all she could about longevity and healthy living.

Bettie passed away on December 11, 2008, at age eighty-five, after suffering a heart attack, but her legacy lives on and only continues to grow over time. She's such an enduring star, in fact, that for years she has been featured on *Forbes* magazine's annual list of top-earning deceased celebrities. In 2016 her estate earned an estimated $11 million—almost double the amount of $6 million in 2011, and placing her ahead of Marilyn Monroe.

Bettie is so iconic that contemporary icons frequently emulate her: Madonna, Katy Perry, Beyoncé, and other stars have borrowed her look for both professional and personal use, and she has been the muse of top fashion designers and countless musicians and artists. Even John Lydon of Public Image Ltd. (formerly known as Johnny Rotten of the Sex Pistols) recorded a song and video called "Bettie Page" for his 2015 album. "She had the courage to do something no one else was doing," he told *Rolling Stone*. "I admired what she was doing . . . so it's a song of admiration."

Bettie's singular influence is evident not only on movie screens, in music videos, and on runways, but in countless present-day women who fashion their style after Bettie in one way or another.

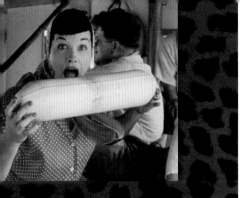

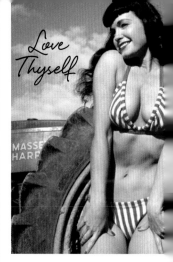

*Love
Thyself*

CHAPTER THREE

*the*

# BOLDNESS

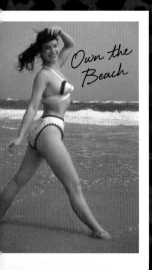

*Own the
Beach*

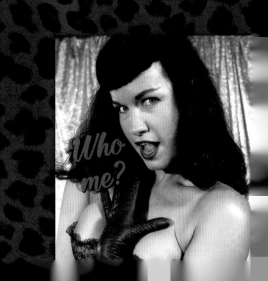

*Who
me?*

"You know why I think people equate me with the sexual revolution? Because I wasn't uptight. As far as nudity and sex was concerned, I did what I felt like doing no matter what other people thought. That's what must make me stand out."

—Bettie Page

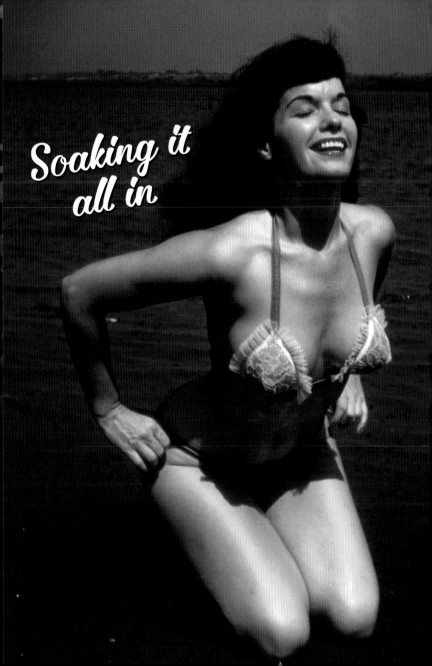

Soaking it all in

*W*HEN PEOPLE COME TO KNOW about Bettie, they usually fall in love in two stages: First they see her photos, somehow somewhere, and they are awed by the specialness and simple-but-powerful beauty that is evident just by looking at her. Pinup photographer and makeup artist Angelica Luna, of San Bernardino, California, first caught sight of Bettie on a boy's T-shirt when she was in high school and was instantly hooked. "I thought she just looked so badass, tough, sexy, and curvaceous! I knew I had to find out who she was."

As it was for Luna, that initial discovery is usually followed by rapid consumption of every possible bit of information about Bettie, along with a gazillion more stunning photos that she took in her short pinup career. When fans learn the details of her life, her losses and risks, and all she went through, the sense of awe deepens tremendously. One of Bettie's defining traits was the sheer amount of courage and confidence she repeatedly displayed, and that's something her female fans in particular call on for strength: "I love her boldness, her ability to put herself out there without fear, and her attitude that seems to say, 'This is how I am, take it or leave it,'" says BrittanyJean. "I am not as bold as I would like to be, and I find myself at times sort of 'channeling' her when I need to be sassy or more forward."

"Bettie inspires me to be a stronger, more confident woman all the time. I catch a lot of comments about how I am built—I'm not as curvy as a lot of other pinup girls, and I have seen some truly heartbreaking words written about how I don't belong or that I'm not built like a 'real woman.' Bettie reminds me to be strong and that I am beautiful and sexy in my own way."

*—BrittanyJean*

This was a woman who continually bucked the odds and convention: at one point a young woman with a college degree living independently in a big city, and ultimately enduring serious pain and disappointment from her failed relationships, infertility, and dashed dreams of silver-screen stardom. She survived child abuse, poverty,

OPPOSITE, CLOCKWISE FROM TOP: Bettie's kind of multitasking • These boots were made for kicking ass! • Jungle Bettie looking fierce in another DIY creation

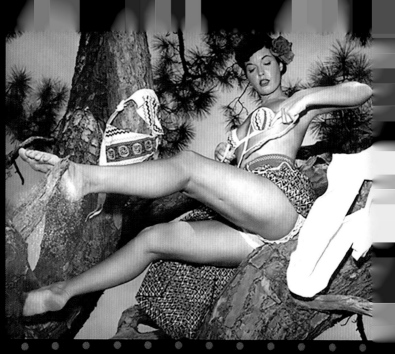

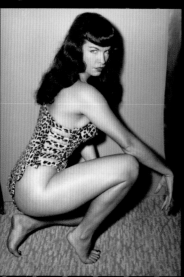

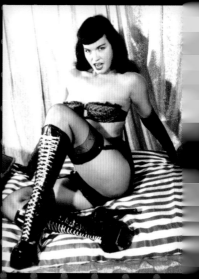

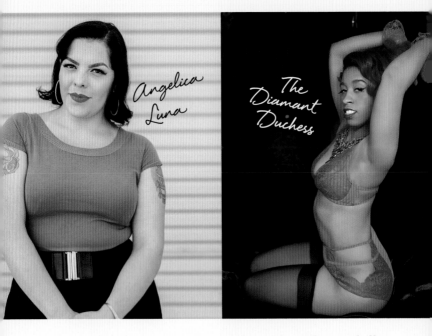

*Angelica Luna*

*The Diamant Duchess*

incest, domestic violence, sexual assault, and mental illness, all before there was any semblance of legal or social support for people facing these issues. And yet she persisted and often thrived despite her circumstances. If ever someone could be described as having grit, it's Bettie. Lots of women have been affected by some of the same issues and view her as a beacon of hope that the human spirit can endure such tragedy and still prevail so purely.

"Bettie Page has inspired me to keep moving forward because she kept going through all her hardships," says the Diamant Duchess, a pinup model and stylist from Atlanta.

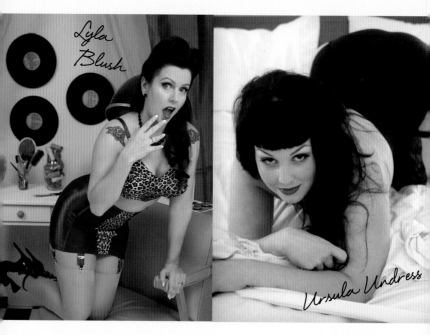

Lyla Blush

Ursula Undress

"The high standard she held for herself and the way she demanded respect from those around her should be a reminder to all women to respect yourself, and don't sell yourself short." To keep that top of mind, Ursula Undress, coowner of the Atlanta School of Burlesque, got a Bettie tattoo on her arm: "I got the tattoo of her to remind myself that she lives in me somewhere, even when I am feeling down. I work very hard to be a vivacious woman that is full of life, and her image reminds me of that."

For some women, Bettie has been a real lifesaver. That is true for model, photographer, and stylist Lyla Blush, of Leesburg, Georgia, who drew strength from Bettie that helped her eventually leave a physically and emotionally abusive seven-year relationship. "She was all that I wanted to be by all appearances—strong, confident, and sexual without feeling shame," Blush recalls. "That all came for me, eventually, and it began with learning of Bettie Page. I am forever grateful to her for that." That influence has trickled down to Blush's two daughters, who she says are strong and independent, and to her son, who has learned to respect women.

# BODY-POSITIVE PIONEER

THROUGH ALL OF HER STRUGGLES, Bettie carried herself with a strong sense of self-acceptance that shone through her photos. Her obvious confidence always stood out and has inspired scores of women over the years in a way than no one else has been able to. Along with general self-confidence, she has done wonders for her fans' body confidence. "Bettie Page helped me love my body—I think that is the most important thing I can take from her," states Jasmin Rodriguez, model, fashion blogger, and editor-in-chief of Vintage-vandalizm.com. "I remember doing my own shoots trying to

OPPOSITE: Bettie's fans often feel validated when they see Bettie's bit of cellulite—and realize she's perfect anyway.

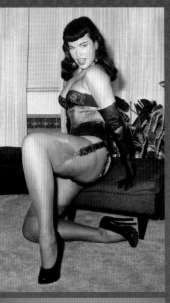

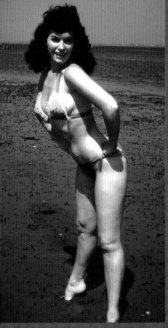

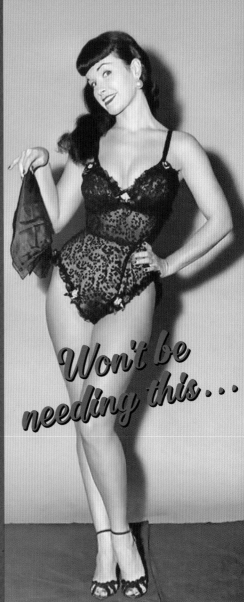

*Won't be needing this . . .*

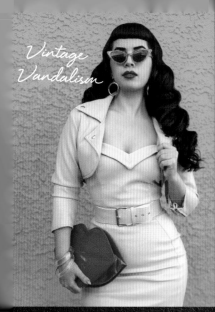

*Vintage Vandalism*

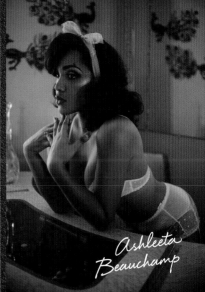

*Ashleeta Beauchamp*

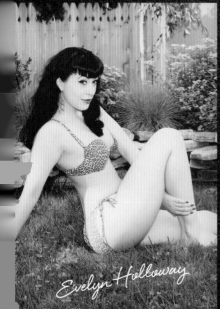

*Evelyn Holloway*

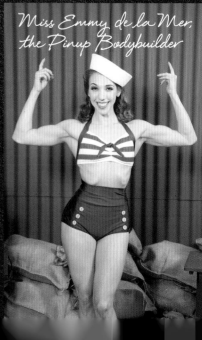

*Miss Emmy de la Mer, the Pinup Bodybuilder*

emulate her poses. She was amazing at posing! You can see her influence in my images." The same goes for pinup model Evelyn Holloway, who used to wonder as a teenager why she wasn't stick-thin like some of her friends. "But when I got into Bettie Page, I thought, 'My idol has curves, so it's okay for me to,'" she recalls. "Now I'm proud of my body."

As you might expect from someone said to have influenced the sexual revolution, Bettie has also served as a prime example that nudity doesn't have to be linked with shame. She maintained that belief even after she became a born-again Christian, saying she didn't believe that God disapproved of nudity because he made Adam and Eve that way. She once remarked that she hoped to be remembered as someone who changed society's perception of nudity in its natural form, and that rare ease she had with her own is one of the most intriguing things about her. She loved to swim or be out in nature sans clothing, and she talked in interviews about hanging around the house naked during her beloved "air baths."

"She seemed so free and is such an example of how to love your body and what you were born with," says Ashleeta Beauchamp, a pinup model and burlesque performer. Of course, Bettie was beyond beautiful, but she had what some would consider imperfections—like fine lines and cellulite—and yet she freely and happily showed herself off anyway. Ashleeta cites Bettie as a major influence on her, especially in "being comfortable during my burlesque performances, being nude without actually feeling nude and just being comfortable with myself. There's just something about her where she appears nude but not naked."

I love Bettie's underdog victory of having been rejected by Ford Modeling Agency and ultimately becoming one of the most iconic models of all time. At five foot five inches and 120 pounds or so, and with an unusually small waist in proportion to her hips, she was shorter and curvier than the typical model, even in the '50s. There is a misconception that models back then had a similar shape to Bettie and Marilyn Monroe, but these icons were actually the exception, rather than the rule. Bettie was an early fan of health food, but she didn't deprive herself and made room for her favorites, like fried chicken and ice cream. She believed that eating is one of life's greatest pleasures.

That doesn't mean she never struggled with her weight or body image. In fact, the main reason Bettie wouldn't allow herself to be shown in photographs or on video after her modeling years was that she was ashamed that she had gained a substantial amount of weight, and she wanted fans to remember her as she was in her pinup years. Though some of my therapist colleagues who specialize in body image might view this as incongruent with Bettie's status as a body positive icon, I view it as a more complex issue. First, her status as a symbol of self-acceptance and body positivity is not based on intellectual ideas, but on the very clear sense of joy and comfort in her body that is evident in her photos.

For many women, that sort of vivid example has a more

> "With all the body shaming out there in the media and online, it is delightful to see more of a body-positivity trend happening. We can thank Bettie for representing that."
>
> — *Miss Emmy de la Mer*

powerful impact than being told to love their bodies. All the experts in the world can't make someone love her body by telling her to. We need visual examples of other women in the very act of loving their bodies—and for lots of women, Bettie is the prototype of that kind of body love. She literally embodies body positivity in her photos, even if she was unhappy with her body at other points in her life, and that doesn't take away from the symbolic value she holds in women's lives. "With all the body shaming out there in the media and online, it is delightful to see more of a body positivity trend happening," says DC-based Miss Emmy de la Mer, also known as the Pinup Bodybuilder. "We can thank Bettie for representing that."

"The thing that inspires me most about Bettie is her no-bullshit attitude. She ran with her interests rather than waiting for someone to tell her what she was doing was okay. Even in the face of public pushback against an art form seen as taboo, Bettie Page was having fun and being herself. I try to approach my art and my life with that same exact attitude."

—*Whittney Chaplin,*
BOSTON-BASED MODEL AND HAIRSTYLIST

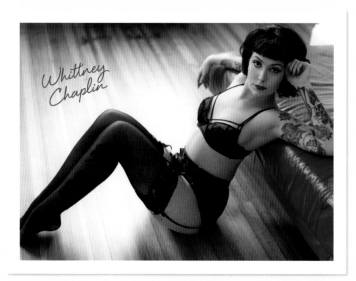

To me, Bettie's weight issues are yet another reminder that she was a real person, as authentic as they come, and that even the pinup queen of the universe experienced the same types of problems the rest of us have. That deserves compassion, rather than judgment, and doesn't negate her impact on her fans' self-confidence. Not to mention that "loving your body" isn't always a realistic goal, and it often gets interpreted as "love how your body looks" even if that isn't the intention. You might not be able to love how your body looks on command, but you *can* find ways to take care of and appreciate your body. So think of it not so much as loving how your body looks (though kudos to you if you do!) but more like focusing on how it feels, what it does, and *showing* love to it by giving it what you know it needs: regular physical activity, solid nutrition, and sufficient rest, to name the very basics.

Body positivity isn't just about weight, either. It's about combating stigma against physical disabilities and creating space and visibility for people who live with them. It's also about fighting body shame in other forms—like the shame associated with women's nude bodies. It's ironic that we talk about how scandalous Bettie's nude photos were in her day, but Facebook and Instagram rigorously censor female nudity. Bettie's own Instagram page was actually suspended temporarily because of a photo in which the nipples were not blurred out enough!

Yet, women are still constantly sexually objectified in ads, magazines, online, and on TV and film. Basically, it seems that sexuality in women is acceptable when it is done to them but not by them, so to speak—when it's forced on them but not when it's initiated by them. That's another major reason that Bettie was and still is such a rarity: you could tell just by looking at her that she alone was in charge of her body and her sexuality, and she wasn't the least bit sorry about it.

The ever-present attempts to control women's bodies in various ways make a particular incident involving Bettie all the more relevant today. During one of many outdoor photo shoots with a camera club, she and the photographers were arrested for public indecency. In court, Bettie boldly declared, "I'm not indecent! I will not plead guilty to it!" And indeed, she didn't—after all the fuss she made, the charge was reduced to disorderly conduct. It is almost unfathomable that before there was any notable movement to reduce shame about women's nudity or to sexually empower women, somehow Bettie just got it and stood up for herself—and by extension, for all of us.

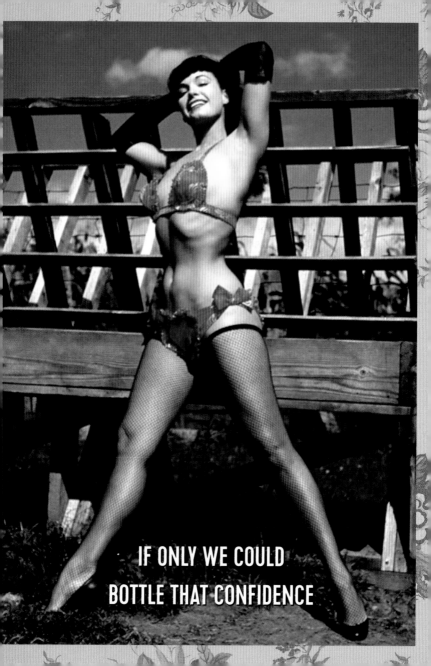

IF ONLY WE COULD
BOTTLE THAT CONFIDENCE

# Diversity on the Pinup Scene

On top of being a playground of beauty, fashion, music, and cool cars, the modern pinup scene is also a stage for social change. Though the original style arose in a time of more explicit racial oppression, the contemporary pinup community is more inclusive and offers women of color an avenue for expression outside the confines of mainstream stereotypes. "It allows me to embrace my femininity, which is often subject to being taken away from women of color because of our non-European features," says pinup model Velvet Wren. But that doesn't mean there isn't much progress still to be made. "With faces like Rita Hayworth, Marilyn Monroe, and Elizabeth Taylor being at the forefront of what the idea of a pinup girl is, women of color tend to have to do more research on what to do with their hair, makeup, and clothes," for example. She and these other groundbreaking gals are widening the lens on what it means to be a pinup.

ASHLEETA: I think there is a misconception that women of color were never part of the pinup community to begin with, or that we didn't exist back then. There were pinup models of color in the early days of pinup, like Lottie the Body, Toni Elling, and Ernestine Terry. They just didn't receive the exposure or opportunities their white counterparts did. A lot of these women doubled as burlesque dancers, but so did a good number of pinups in that day. There are problems that I believe have carried over to the present: the lack of opportunity and the idea of tokenism—for example, a company might feel like they don't need to book more than one model of color for a shoot. I think the best way to address this issue is to communicate openly and listen to women of color in the pinup community without getting defensive. There's enough room for all of us.

**THE DIAMANT DUCHESS:** Overall, the pinup scene is very welcoming. With its growth in recent years through social media and pop culture, I'm hoping the cultural diversity will continue to grow as well. There are so many people with various backgrounds and views who offer different ways of seeing things and promote a sense of inclusivity.

**ANGELIQUE NOIRE:** I am always very conscious of how I present myself in photos, especially if I am wearing lingerie or swimwear. As a black woman, society has had this stigma that labels us as "overly sexual" or "vulgar," and I don't want to play into those stereotypes. Smiling is my favorite expression, and I know the power it holds to balance an image. I often think of the playful images of Bettie and imagine how I can project elements of her influence.

**VELVET WREN:** The pinup community is diverse, and there are a lot of women of color redefining what pinups look like. I am the admin and owner of Pinups of Colour, and I get messages every day from women thanking me for posting them or introducing them to a model they can relate to. It makes me happy and truly grateful to be a part of this community and contribute to women of color seeing themselves as pinups and vintage enthusiasts without shame. I feel that the neo-pinup revolution is also very inclusive in embracing body positivity and dismantling the ideas of ableism and gender as limits in pinup. As with every movement, there is always more room for growth.

# the
# BODY

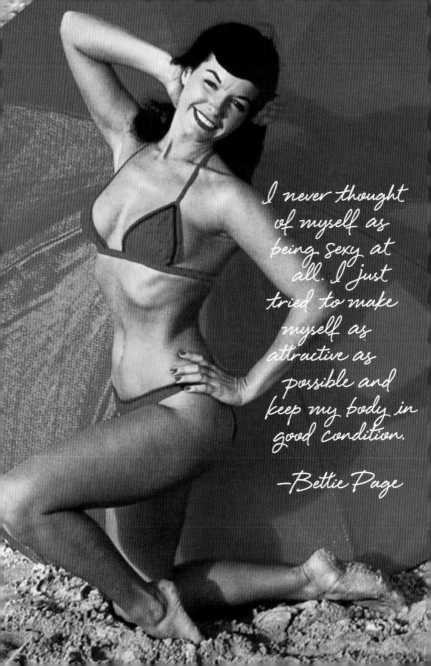

*I never thought of myself as being sexy at all. I just tried to make myself as attractive as possible and keep my body in good condition.*

—Bettie Page

MONG THE INFINITE REASONS Bettie fans are awestruck by her: She just looks like the epitome of health and vibrancy in her photos, with glowing skin and more muscle definition than was common for women of her day. There is good reason for that. Bettie was the rare woman in that era who worked out—in a New York City gym, no less!

Back then, women might use "reducing machines" designed to slim the body with minimal physical exertion, according to Natalia Petrzela, PhD, a history professor at the New School in New York City, and the fitness historian for Well+Good. These contraptions "were often adjacent to beauty salons or located in private homes—not in gyms, which were still considered the preserve of sweaty, grunting men and entirely inappropriate for respectable ladies who often kept their high heels on during a reducing session." Not our Bettie! It seems she was right there with those sweaty, grunting guys putting in some real work.

She loved to swim, go dancing or walking, play sports, and do calisthenics. I'm also convinced that she was doing yoga. These various forms of exercise often showed up in Bettie's photos—for instance a Camel Pose or Plow Pose here, a squat or a lunge or an ab crunch there. This sparked

THE BODY

my idea to create the Bettie Page Fitness workouts that are inspired by Bettie in several different ways. Each move in the workouts is based on a specific photo of Bettie, with an emphasis on the amazing balance, perfect posture, and core strength Bettie displayed. I don't encourage women (or myself) to try to get the "Bettie body," since her shape was largely determined by genetics. And while her body was undoubtedly spectacular, there are many different types of beautiful bodies, and not solely because of how they look.

If you study Bettie's movements through hundreds or thousands of poses, you'll notice that the great majority of them are big, open, expansive, and outward—you can tell she was unafraid to take up her rightful space in the world, both physically and figuratively. By emulating her body postures, we are harnessing that same energy and cultivating those traits. They are what scientists now call "Power Poses," and they have been found to reduce stress, improve body image, and increase confidence. I've purposely included lots of power poses in the Bettie Page Fitness workouts, which also happen to be the first-ever body-positive fitness videos.

Like Bettie's fitness sampler platter, a solid exercise practice should include strength-based moves, cardio, and flexibility training of some sort. All types of movement are generally a plus for the body, increasing circulation and helping to keep things in working order, but the different types of exercise provide specific benefits too: Strength training builds muscle mass and improves bone health; cardiovascular exercise is especially beneficial for heart health; and yoga, Pilates, and Tai Chi can boost flexibility, balance, and core strength.

Just about any type of physical activity will lift your mood. Not only does exercise increase feel-good chemicals released by the brain, such as pain-relieving endorphins and mood-regulating neurotransmitters, but it also gives a sense of accomplishment from challenging yourself and doing something kind for your body. It also reduces internal inflammation caused by illness, unhealthy lifestyle choices, and external toxins, such as air pollution and pesticides.

You don't have to be a purist and get each type of exercise separately. Some workouts, like the ones I've created for you below, offer two or all of these components, or you can combine them however you'd like. For example, after a strength or cardio workout, you might cool down with a ten- or fifteen-minute yoga flow or Pilates practice. Some types of yoga actually qualify as both strengthening and flexibility exercise, so you could take a power yoga class online or in person if you want to knock out both in one pop. Or, if you hate the idea of doing straight cardio for an extended amount of time or just don't have the energy for it on a given day, you could instead insert some cardio bursts between moves in your strength workout.

And don't think you're limited to straight-up, regimented exercise. Take a cue from Bettie and go dancing (in the privacy of your home is fine!), swimming, or hiking to keep things fun and fresh.

# Maintaining a Body-Positive Focus

Keep this in mind when you do these workouts:

- Aim to infuse them with the same sense of joy and strength you see when you look at Bettie's poses.

- Have gratitude for the ability to move and take care of your body, and thank yourself for making the time to do it.

- Notice the sensations you feel in each move, and play around with variations to see what works best for your body, whether just for today or in general.

- Have fun exploring each exercise, and when you wobble or struggle with a certain move, take it as a reminder that you're challenging yourself, learning something new, and resisting that pesky perfectionism that can ruin the party.

- Instead of a weight or appearance goal, try setting goals based on achievement: Work up to twelve-pound dumbbells versus eight-pound ones, for example, or nail a headstand for ten seconds.

# the PINUP POWER POSE *workout*

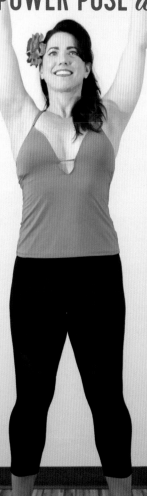

Adapted from my *Bettie Page Fitness: Total Body Strength & Cardio* workout DVD.

- Starting with the first two moves, do two back-to-back (except the two stretches at the end), for up to three sets each, before moving onto the next pair of moves.

- A set of five- to twelve-pound dumbbells is recommended for moves 1, 3, and 5.

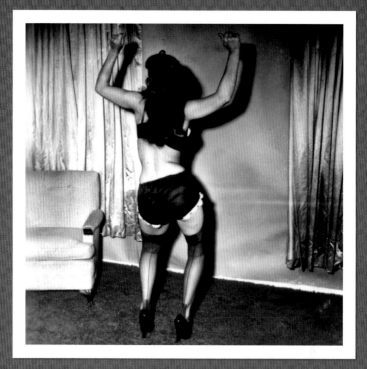

# Squat with Overhead Press

Stand with feet slightly wider than hip-width apart, holding a dumb-bell in each hand with arms extended to sides and bent 90 degrees in a goalpost position (like Bettie's as shown here). Lower into a squat position and pause briefly. Return to standing as you press the weights overhead (until arms are straight) and rise onto your toes. Hold for one count and then return to starting position and repeat. Do 10 to 15 reps per set.

# Star Jump

Stand with feet hip-width
apart and lower into a
half-squat with your arms
bent in front of you and
hands around shoulder
level (like you're at the top
of a biceps hammer curl).
Jump up and out into a
Star Pose, with legs wide
apart and arms out-
stretched straight to the
sides (as shown by Bettie).
Do 20 per set.

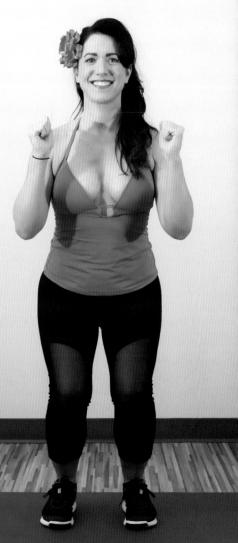

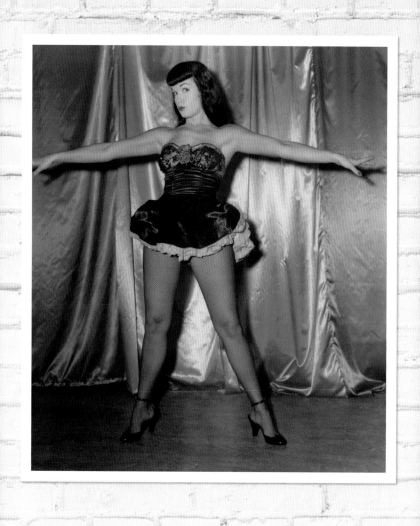

# Rear Lunge to Knee-Up and Bicep Curl

Stand with feet hip-width apart and hold a dumbbell in each hand. Step your right leg back into a lunge, making sure that your left knee doesn't come past your toes

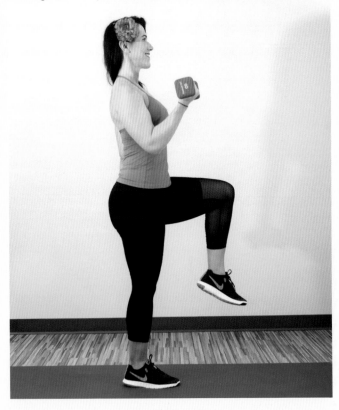

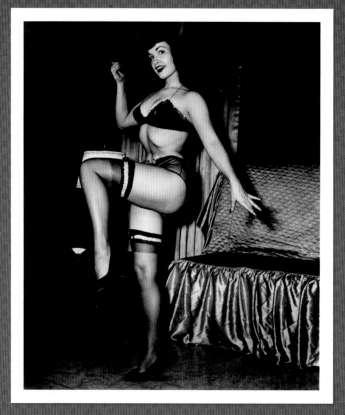

(to protect your knees). In a continuous motion, push off the right
foot to return to an upright position and tap the toes to the floor
before bringing the right knee up in front of you until your right thigh
is roughly parallel to the floor. As you lift the knee, do a biceps curl
with the left arm, then lower the arm as you lower your right foot to
the floor, tapping it lightly before lunging back again for the next rep.
Complete a total of 12 reps on each side.

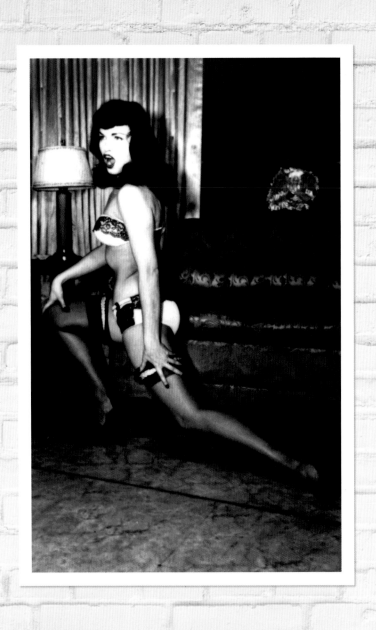

# Jumping Lunge

Stand with feet hip-width apart and step the right foot back into a lunge. Keeping your core tight, jump up and switch legs midair to land in a lunge with the left leg back. As you switch legs, extend one arm (either left or right is okay, whichever feels best) in front of you and the other behind you, as shown, and switch the arms as you jump to switch legs. Repeat for a total of 20 lunges per set.

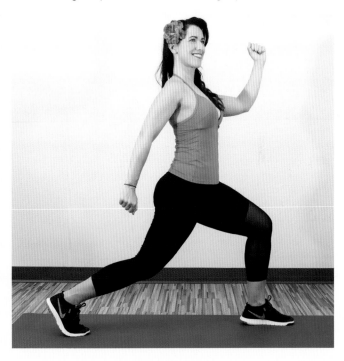

# Narrow Squat with Heel Lift and Upright Row

Stand with feet together or just 1 or 2 inches apart (see what feels best to your knees in this move), holding dumbbells in front of you at your thighs. Pull your shoulder blades back and avoid slouching. Contract your abs and butt and lower to a squat, letting the weights come down in front of your knees as you go. At the bottom, lift your heels as you bring the weights into an upright row. Pause briefly before lowering your heels and weights as you return to standing. That's one rep; do a total of 10 to 15 per set.

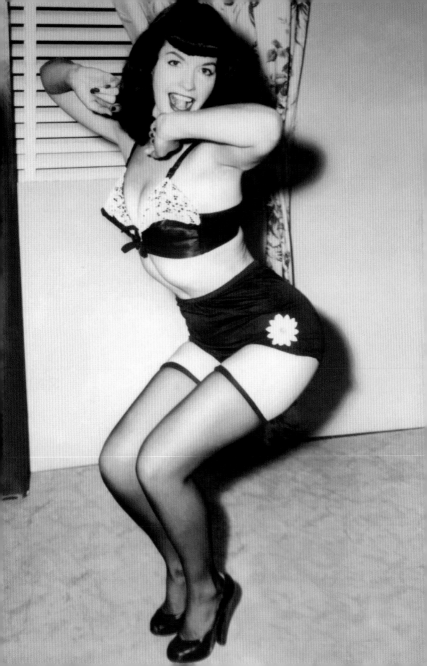

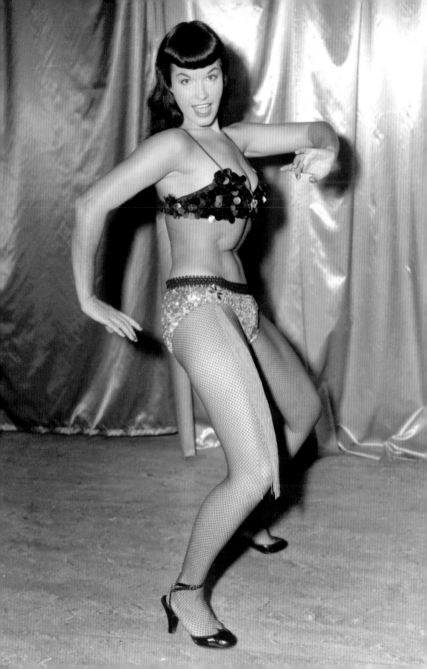

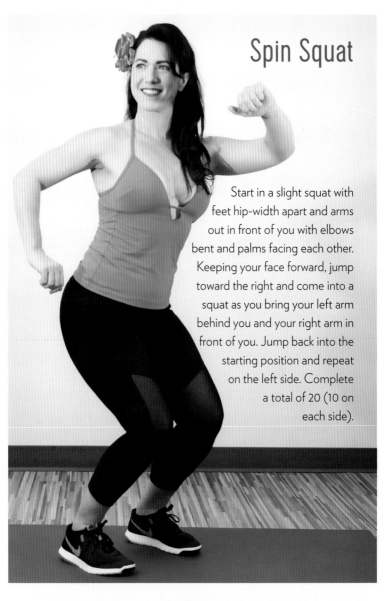

# Spin Squat

Start in a slight squat with feet hip-width apart and arms out in front of you with elbows bent and palms facing each other. Keeping your face forward, jump toward the right and come into a squat as you bring your left arm behind you and your right arm in front of you. Jump back into the starting position and repeat on the left side. Complete a total of 20 (10 on each side).

# Cross-Leg Diagonal Crunch

Rest the outer edge of your right foot just above your left knee, bring your hands behind your head or ears, and extend your elbows out. Think of reaching your left shoulder toward your right knee as you crunch in that direction. Do a total of 10 to 15 reps, then do that same number of little pulses at the top of the crunch. Repeat on the other side.

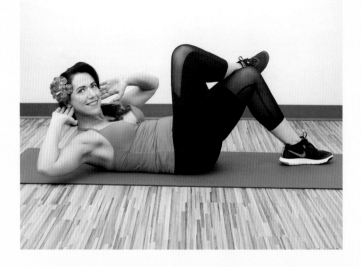

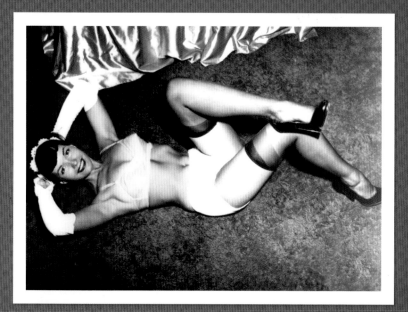

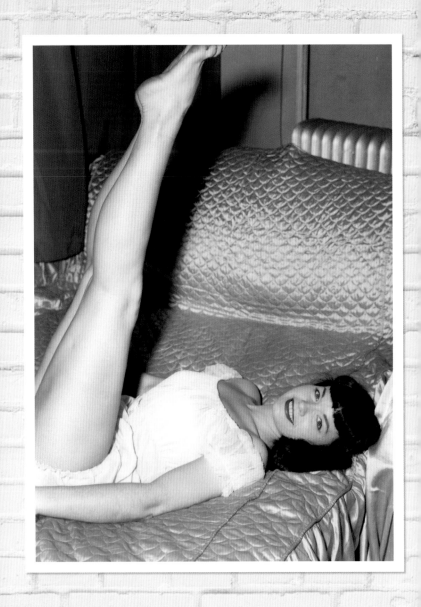

# Hip Lift and Toe Touch

Lie back with your arms on the floor at your sides, and lift your legs straight up. (If your hamstrings are tight, bend the knees slightly.) First, lift the hips a couple of inches off the floor and then bring them back down, quickly, repeating 10 to 15 times. Next, with legs still extended, keep your hips grounded as you reach your hands as high as you can toward your feet and pulse up and down 10 to 15 times.

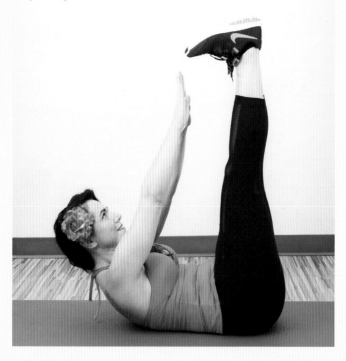

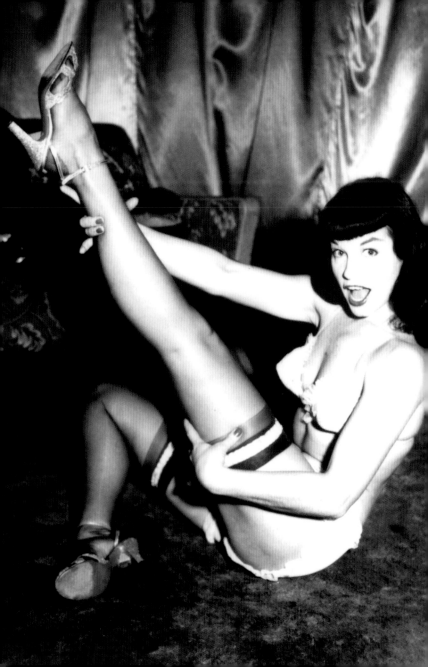

# Heron Stretch

This hamstring stretch is inspired by yoga's Heron pose. While seated on the floor, bend your left knee and bring it in front of you, resting the outer leg on the floor as shown. Extend the right leg straight up in front of you (again, okay to bend the knee if you have tight hamstrings) and hold with one or both hands. Hold the stretch as you breathe in and out slowly and deeply at least 3 times, then switch sides and repeat. (Repeat a couple times on each side if your hamstrings are super-tight.)

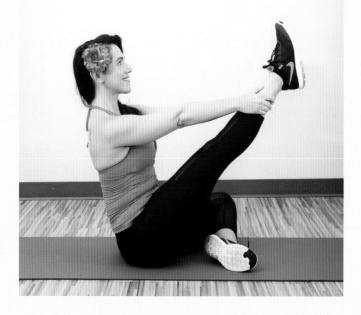

# Hip Lift Stretch

From a Heron stretch, keep your left leg where it is and bring your right leg behind you to rest the inner leg on the floor, with knee bent and heel near your butt. Your left foot should be near your right knee. Plant your hands a few inches behind your butt and press into them while lifting your hips up and forward until you feel a stretch. Hold for at least 3 full breaths. Optional: Take it into a yoga twist when you plant your butt, by grabbing your left knee with your right hand and turning to look over your left shoulder.

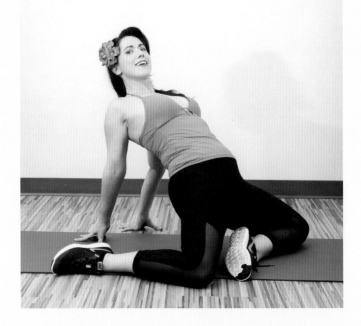

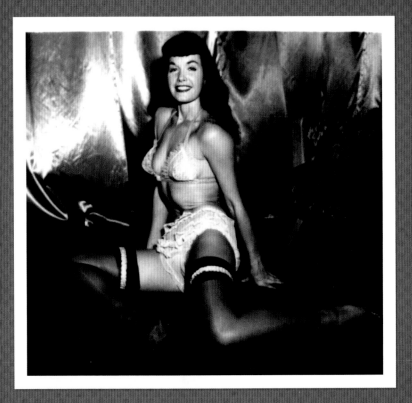

After you finish the Heron and Hip Lift stretches on one side, do both on the other side.

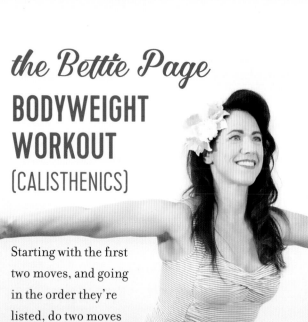

# the Bettie Page
# BODYWEIGHT
# WORKOUT
## (CALISTHENICS)

Starting with the first
two moves, and going
in the order they're
listed, do two moves
back-to-back for
up to four sets
each (except for
the two stretches
at the end) before
moving onto the next
pair of moves.

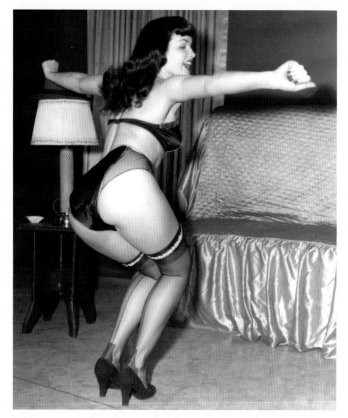

# Narrow Squat with Arms Extension

Standing with feet together or a couple inches apart, make a fist with your hands and bring them together in front of your chest. Lower into a squat as you extend your arms straight out to each side. Pause briefly, then rise to standing as you bring your arms back in and fists together in front of you. Do 15 to 20 reps per set.

# Good Morning

Standing with feet hip-width apart, bring your hands behind your head and extend your elbows out to the sides. Contract your core and butt and keep your back strong as you hinge forward from the hips with a flat back (and slight bend in the knees, if needed) until your back is roughly parallel to the floor. Keeping your core engaged and back flat, contract your glutes to bring yourself back to standing.

Do a total of 15 to 20 reps per set.

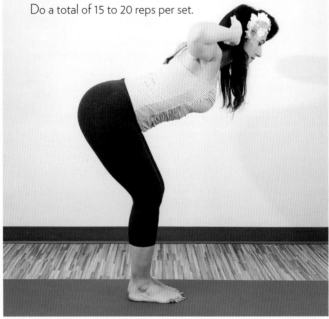

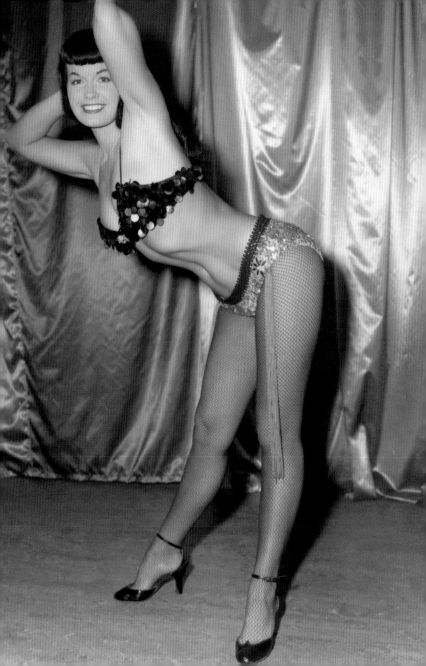

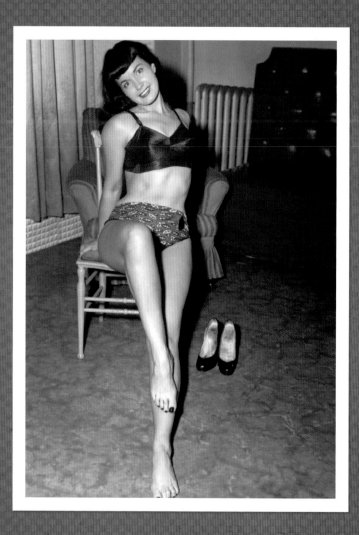

# Seated Leg Extension

Sit up straight on the edge of a chair or another sturdy surface of a similar height, and place your hands just behind you on it. Lift your right leg a few inches off the floor and flex your foot with knee bent, then extend the leg straight in front of you and pause for one count before returning to bent knee. Straighten and bend 15 to 20 times, then repeat on the other side.

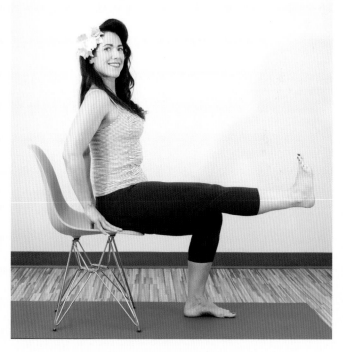

# Push-Up

Start with your knees on the floor and arms straight with palms flat on the floor under your shoulders. Bend your elbows while keeping them close to your sides, and lower your upper body until your chest hovers a few inches above the floor. If you prefer full push-ups on your toes, go for it! Do 15 to 20 reps per set.

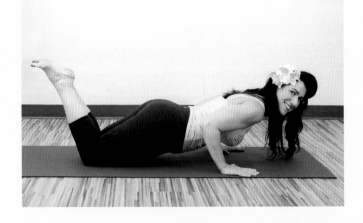

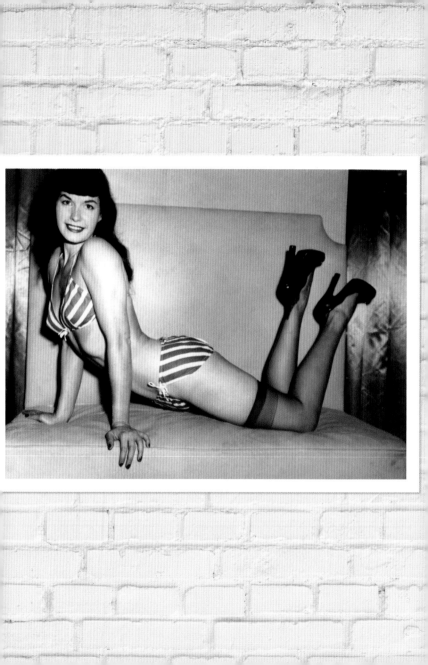

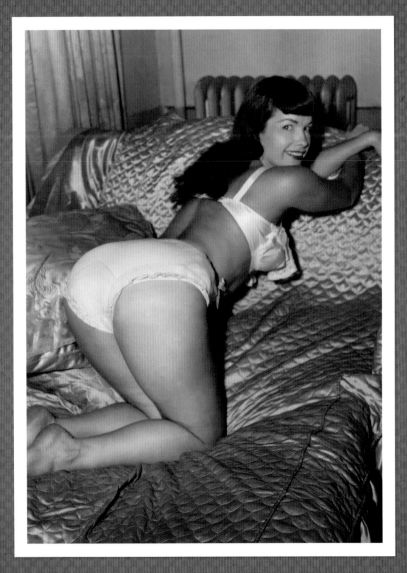

# Glute Kickbacks

Get on all fours and bring your forearms down to rest on the floor and clasp your hands. Extend the right leg straight back and up behind you, then pause for one count before returning to starting position. Repeat 15 to 20 times before switching to the other side to repeat.

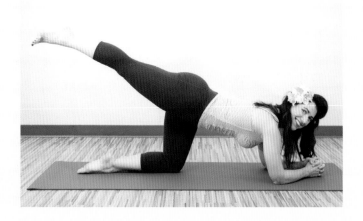

# Table with Leg Extension

Start in what I call "Mudflap Girl" position, seated on the floor with knees bent and palms planted on the floor a few inches behind you with fingertips pointing toward you. Press into the hands and squeeze your butt as you come up into reverse table position. Lift one leg straight out or up if desired, and pause for one count before you lower your butt halfway down and squeeze and press to lift again. Do that 15 to 20 times per side for each set.

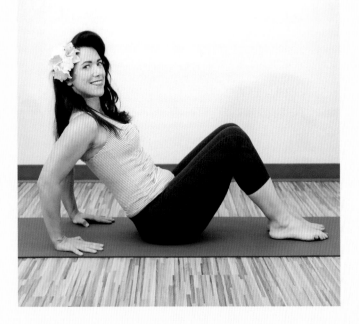

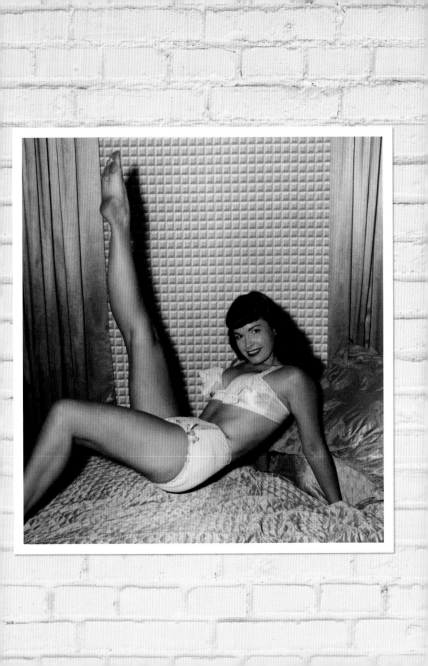

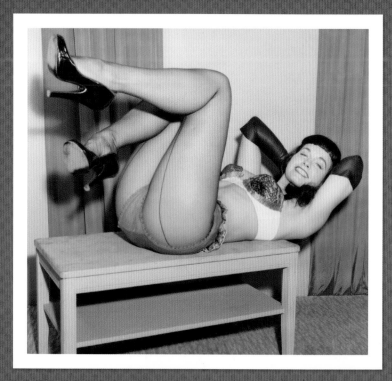

# Bicycle Crunch

Lie on the floor and bring your knees in toward your chest and hands behind your head with elbows out to the sides. Extend your left leg out in front of you at a 45-degree angle (not as low if it hurts your lower back) as you turn your upper body to the right, angling your left elbow toward your bent right knee. Then switch legs and do the same thing toward the left. That's one rep. Do 10 to 15 per set.

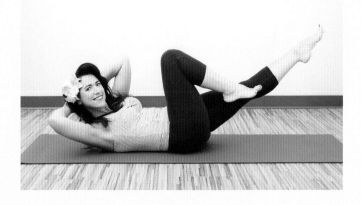

# Knee Drop

Lie on your back and bring your knees in toward your chest with legs together. Lower your knees to the right as far as your lower back will allow without pain (as far as to the floor). Return briefly to center, then lower your knees to the left. That's one rep. Do 10 to 15 per set.

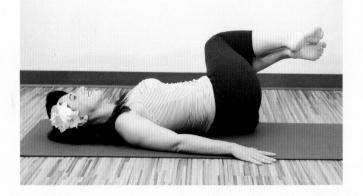

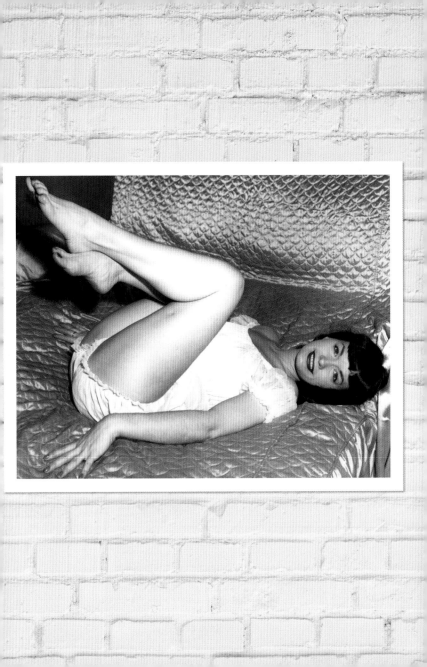

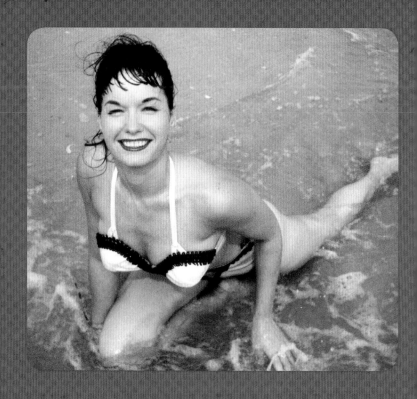

# Pigeon Pose

Start on all fours, then slide the left leg straight back behind you (and walk your hands back as you do, until they are on either side of your knee), making sure that the top of your left foot is resting on the floor to protect your knee. Wiggle your right foot out from under the leg and bring it over toward the left until your right heel is roughly under your left hip. You might feel enough of a stretch there or, for a deeper stretch, you can either walk your hands back closer toward your body or walk them farther out in front of you and fold over the front leg and rest on your elbows. Hold there as you take 10 slow, deep breaths in and out. Then do the next stretch before you do a Pigeon Pose on the other side.

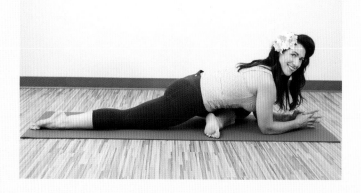

# Yoga Twist

From a Pigeon Pose, keep your right leg where it is, but tilt over toward the right so you can bring your left leg back to the front and around, placing your left foot on the floor just outside your right knee. Place your right hand on the outside of your left knee, and your left hand a few inches behind your butt (flat or on fingertips, whichever feels best to you). Keeping your left butt cheek planted on the floor, lift your torso as you press your hand into your knee, turn to the right, and look past your left shoulder. Hold there for 5 full breaths, lifting as you inhale and deepening the twist as you exhale. Come down and return to all fours, then move into a Pigeon Pose with the left knee in front, followed by the twist on that side.

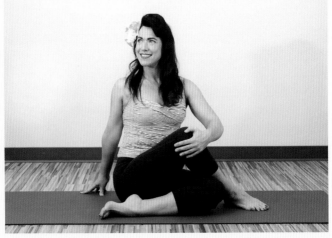

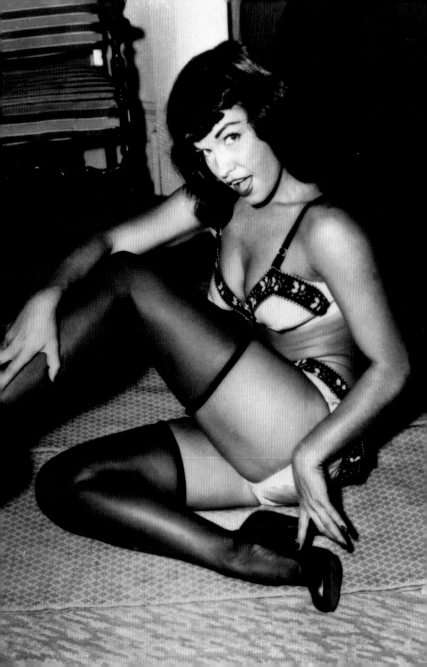

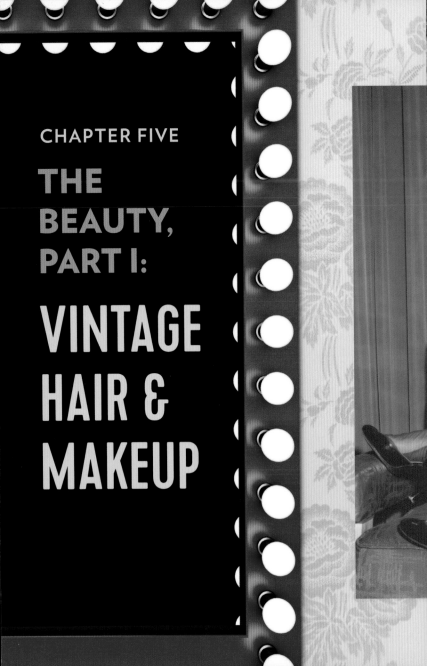

CHAPTER FIVE

# THE BEAUTY, PART I:

# VINTAGE HAIR & MAKEUP

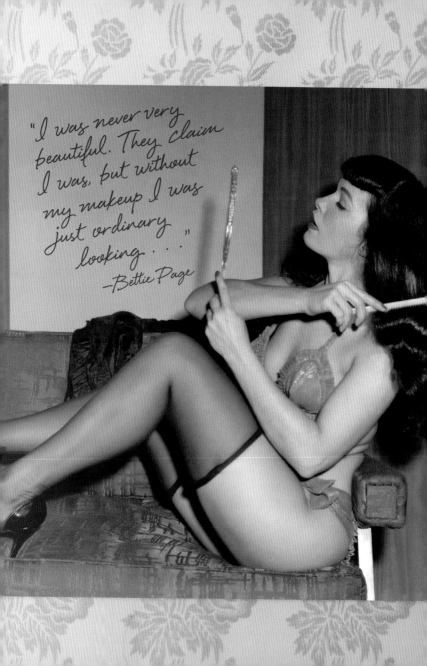

"I was never very beautiful. They claim I was, but without my makeup I was just ordinary looking . . ."
—Bettie Page

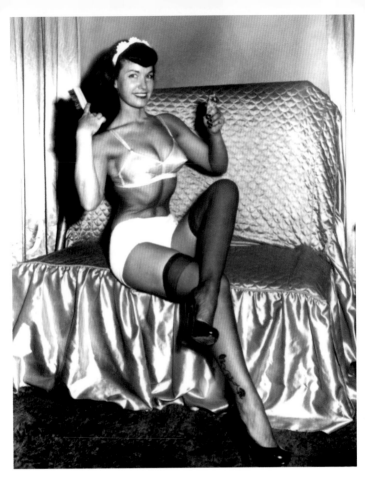

Her unique style varied little
throughout her modeling career,
and yet it never gets old!

**W**ITH HER JET-BLACK HAIR AND EDGY VIBE, Bettie sharply stood out from her sunnier contemporaries like Jayne Mansfield, Marilyn Monroe, and Rita Hayworth. She was, and is, a welcome alternative to the blonde bombshell ideal for plenty of women who don't fit that mold. Her unique style varied little throughout her modeling career, and yet it never gets old! Bettie thought she looked plain without makeup, but she kept it basic—usually just red lips, a little black eyeliner, and brow pencil, which she always did herself. When she got older, her absolute essentials for public outings were brow pencil and lipstick. Ironically, she didn't do the winged eyeliner that is such a hallmark of the pinup look and which usually accompanies Bettie bangs these days. (See sidebar, pages 152–155, for makeup.)

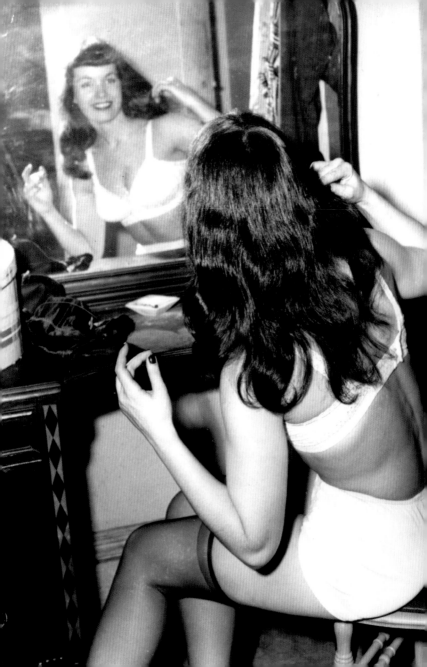

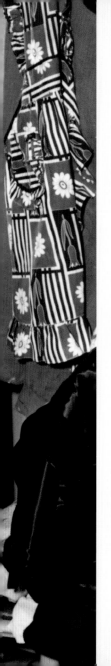

Nor did she wear victory rolls or other common pinup hairstyles. Besides the very occasional ponytail, headband, or hair flower, her hair always had a similar look. (That doesn't mean it was easy—Mark Mori, the director of Bettie's documentary, told me she was constantly running late because she was such a perfectionist about her hair!) She hit on what worked for her and ran with it, and that consistency has no doubt helped to solidify the iconic nature of her signature image. For the rest of us, though, it's nice to have a few go-to alternatives to change it up sometimes. Check out these expert how-tos (by pinup models who often do their own styling à la Queen Bettie!) on glamourous waves, faux Bettie bangs, plus a few additional pinup styles for variation.

# VICTORY ROLLS

**STYLIST AND MODEL**: Meghi Misfit
**PHOTOGRAPHER**: Mikey Martinez

Unless you have naturally curly hair that does what you need it to without much effort (lucky!), setting curls and waves is a key staple of pinup hairstyles. You will generally set your hair the same way for various types of wavy and curly styles, and then you will shape it accordingly. In the Vintage Glamour Wave style shown later in this section (page 135), the stylist shaped the waves a specific way and used clips to achieve that particular 'do, but for less sculpted styles, you can skip the clips and just use your fingers to manipulate hair into the overall shape and direction you're going for after you set the curls.

For this Victory Rolls style, the stylist used a curling iron, but you can play with different methods of setting yours—like hot rollers or a wet set using foam rollers—and settle on the one that works best for your hair. While it may seem like a lot to learn, worry not: You don't have to be a beauty wiz to master these looks, but you will need a healthy dose of patience.

Said to be named for a "victory maneuver" performed by World World II fighter planes, this style that was popularized in the 1940s remains a winner among modern pinups.

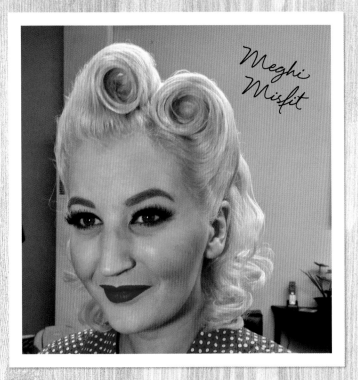

*Meghi Misfit*

## supplies needed

- Gel or setting lotion
- 1/2- or 3/4-inch curlers or curling iron
- Rattail comb
- Double-prong clip

- Hairspray
- Smoothing brush
- Pomade
- Bobby pins

# how to

**Step 1:** Apply gel or setting lotion to damp hair, and set hair using your preferred method. (Be sure to dry hair thoroughly prior to using any heated styling tool!) You will need a ½- or ¾-inch curl for short- to mid-length hair, and you can use up to 1-inch for longer hair, if preferred. Working with 1-inch sections of hair at a time, hold curlers or iron horizontally and roll downward. (For top and sides, roll under in the direction away from the part on either side. For back of hair, roll back and down.)

Leave hot rollers in for at least an hour. If using a curling iron, after you release each curl, pin it into place with a double-prong clip and let cool as shown here. For this style, you might find that working with "day-old" hair holds the shape better. If so, do this one the day after washing.

**Step 2:** Section hair from the top of the head to behind each ear on both sides of the head.

**Step 3:** Starting on the first side section, take 1-inch subsections and tease the base of the hair on both sides. Spray with hairspray. Repeat for the remaining parts of this section.

**Step 4:** Gather all subsections together and smooth the outside of the whole section with a brush. Smooth some pomade on the section and spray with hairspray.

**Step 5:** Pin-curl the section by rolling from the tip down. Pin in place. (Try to hide the pins as much as possible!)

First roll finished!

**Step 6:** Tease the other side section the same way.

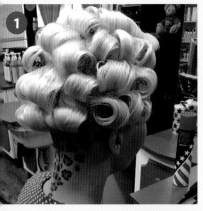
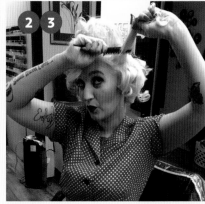
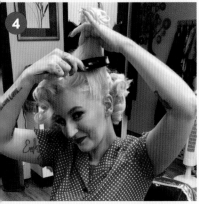
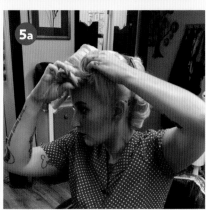
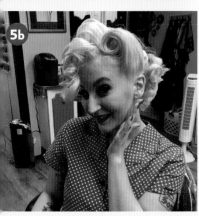
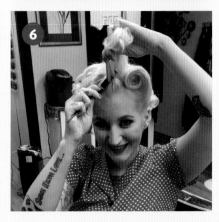

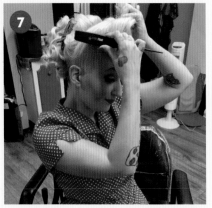
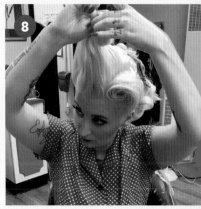
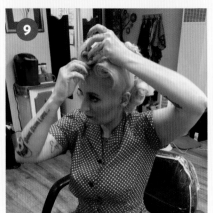
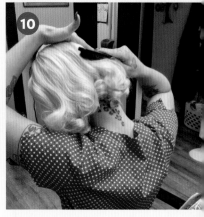

**Step 7:** Smooth the section with a brush, pomade, and hairspray.

**Step 8:** Roll from the tip down to the base and next to the other roll.

**Step 9:** Pin in place.

**Step 10:** Brush out the curls in back of the hair. Spray with hairspray.

All done!

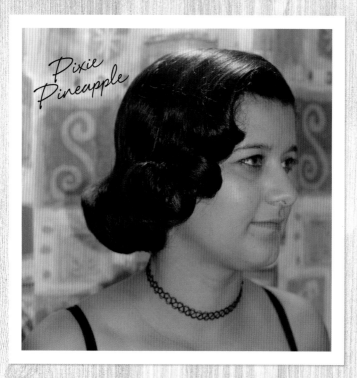

*Pixie Pineapple*

# THE VINTAGE GLAMOUR WAVE

**STYLIST AND PHOTOGRAPHER**: Lyla Blush
**MODEL**: Pixie Pineapple

"Skill level doesn't have to be high, but understanding, persistence, and practice are needed for this style."

—LYLA BLUSH, *stylist and photographer*

## supplies needed

- ○ **Gel or setting lotion**
- ○ **1/2- or 3/4-inch curlers or curling iron**
- ○ **Rattail comb**
- ○ **Pomade**

- ○ **Duckbill clips**
- ○ **Hairspray**
- ○ **Smoothing brush**
- ○ **Bobby pins**

## how to

**Step 1:** Set hair using your preferred method.

**Step 2:** Remove curlers. For the "brush out," use a rattail comb. Part hair to the side, and begin to comb from the part down to the ends, combing over your hand to promote an under-curl. You can reinforce the under-curl by combing from under, forming a nice perfect wave and curl.

**Step 3:** Apply a small amount of pomade to smooth flyaways. You will use a comb to form a wave in the front, then clip the hair into place there and around your head as shown. (Note: If your hair is longer, you will have more waves to clip and hold into place.) If you want a smooth wave in the front, you can form and clip without teasing.

If you would like an elevated wave curl in front, proceed straight to backcombing the top bang section of your hair.

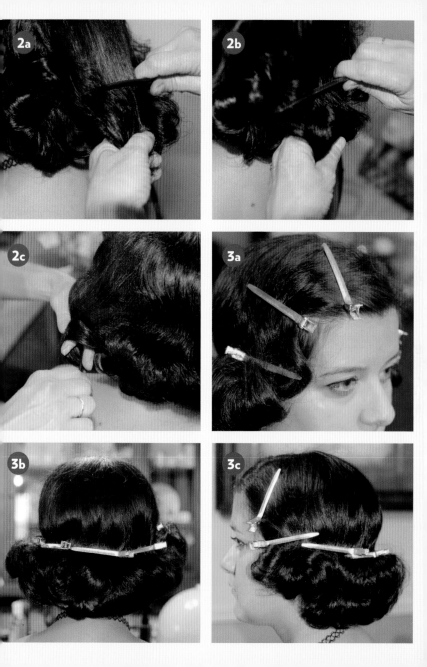

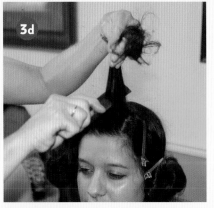

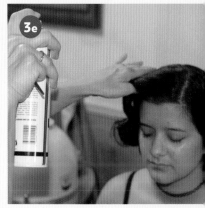

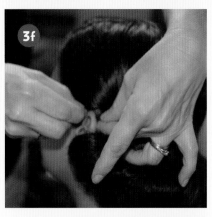

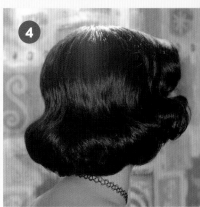

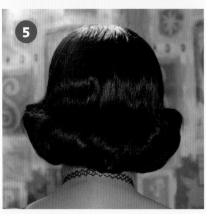

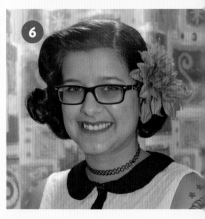

Divide the section into three parts, spray a bit of hairspray, and backcomb or "rat" each section. It will look a mess, but don't worry! Next, you will smooth it over with your smoothing brush (taking care not to undo all the backcombing) to produce a wave next to your face, then clip it into place. Lightly spray your whole head with hairspray.

**Step 4:** Wait at least 15 to 20 minutes, then remove clips and do your final smoothing and shaping of your hair, spraying with hairspray when you're satisfied. I find it easier to accept what my hair has chosen to do at this point to not overdo the 'do. You can smooth one side behind your ear and pin.

**Step 5:** All done! You should have sleek and shiny waves. This style takes practice, so be patient if it takes a few times to perfect to your liking.

**Step 6:** As a final touch, add a hair flower in the area near your bobby pin, apply your favorite lipstick, and you'll be pinup glamour ready!

# FAUX BETTIE BANGS

One thing that makes Bettie-style bangs so eye-catching is that they are quite extreme compared to other types of bangs, since they require cutting into such a large section of hair. And if you know the pain of growing out bangs, go ahead and quadruple that for growing these babies out. Plenty of Bettie Babes have happily made the cut and love it, however, others might long for the look but don't want to make such a drastic commitment. Lucky for us, there's a thing called Clip-In Bettie Bangs. Made with 100 percent human hair, these faux bangs come in different colors and can also be dyed to blend with your hair color. After setting your hair and brushing out your curls, just strategically pin back your hair in the front and clip the bangs in.

Jessica Batiste, the owner of Classy Rebel and maker of Clip-In Bettie Bangs™, wearing her clever creation

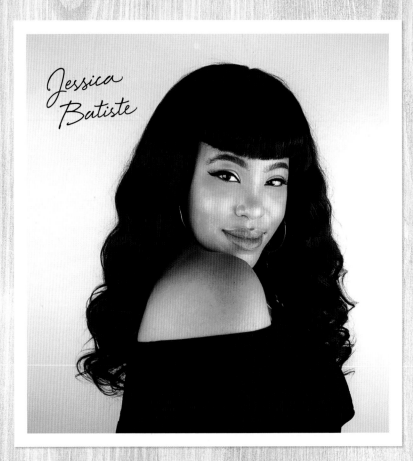

Jessica
Batiste

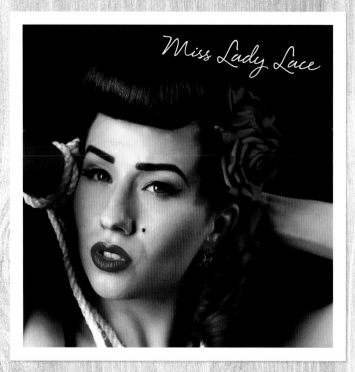

Miss Lady Lace

## BUMPER BANGS

Another way to fake it is with Bettie-style bumper bangs.
You can style these without the doughnut, but using it adds
much more ease and instant volume. Angelica Luna, photographer and stylist at Strawberry D'Lish Pinups, offers
these tips.

# supplies needed

- ○ **Foam doughnut bun in your hair color**
- ○ **Rattail comb**
- ○ **Hairspray**
- ○ **Bobby pins**

# how to

**Step 1:** Cut doughnut bun in half to make one long foam roll.

**Step 2:** For faux bangs, take a section of hair from the forehead going back to roughly the middle of the top of your head; comb to smooth, then spray with hairspray. (If you need extra volume to ensure full coverage over the foam roll, tease and smooth the section before spraying.)

**Step 3:** Place the foam roll under the front hair section, starting at the ends, and roll tightly toward the forehead. Stop in the middle of the forehead, bending slightly on each side in the form of a U shape, and secure each side with bobby pins.

**Step 4:** Your hair will be in the center of the foam roll so you'll want to carefully spread the hair evenly around the rest of the foam to cover it well. Spray with hairspray to hold.

# PINUP STYLES
# FOR TEXTURED HAIR

**STYLIST AND MODEL**: The Diamant Duchess
**PHOTOGRAPHER**: Billy Hawkins Photography

"One great thing about having curly or natural hair is that with the natural thickness and girth, no teasing is required," according to pinup model and stylist the Diamant Duchess. "Hairstyles that often require big-hair teasing can be done much more easily" and with fewer tools. Below she offers a couple of basic styles you can start practicing.

## supplies needed (for both styles)

○ Pomade, styling gel,
   or mousse

○ Bobby pins and a hair tie

○ Scarf

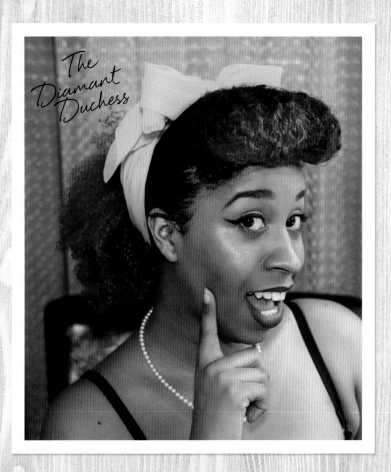

The Diamant Duchess

Bettie Bumper Bangs

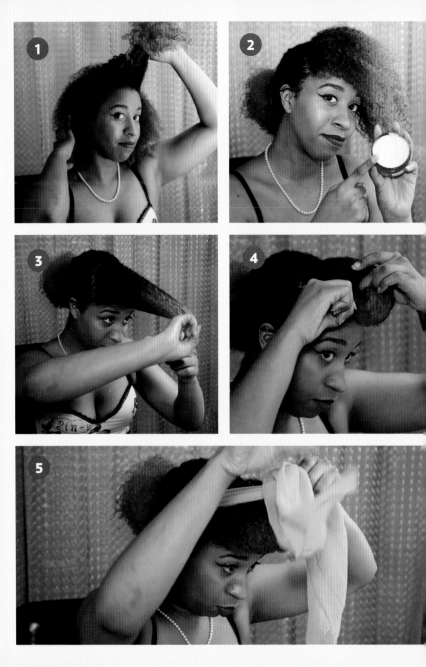

# *how to*

**Step 1:** Start with clean hair, and section off the bang area. As a rough guide, use the edges of your eyebrows as parameters for where to section off the hair. This is how much hair I usually work with for this style.

**Step 2:** Tie back the rest of your hair so it won't get in the way, and apply your favorite pomade, styling gel, or mousse (I prefer pomade) for control and to tame flyaways.

**Step 3:** Now grab the front section and use two fingers as guidance to start rolling your hair toward your forehead.

**Step 4:** Roll it as tight as you can and as close to your head as possible, then grab your bobby pins and start securing your roll on each side, adjusting your bangs as you go.

**Step 5:** When you have your bangs adjusted to your preference, grab a scarf and tie it around your head.

And *voilà*!!!

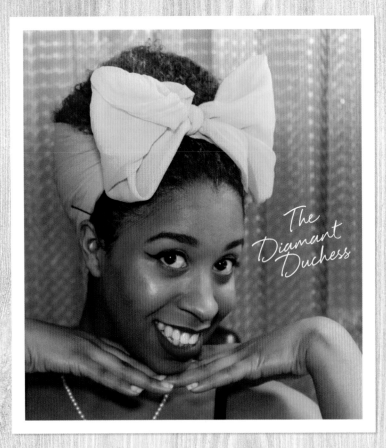

The Diamant Duchess

## The 1960s Bouffant

Though this one became popular slightly after Bettie's modeling era, it is nonetheless a great—and easy!—style to have in your pinup toolbox.

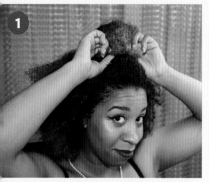
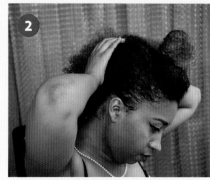
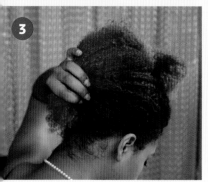
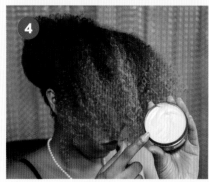

## *how to*

**Step 1:** Starting with clean hair, section off part of the top of your hair. This does not have to be perfect.

**Step 2:** Grab your favorite pomade, styling gel, or mousse, and start smoothing the sides of your hair.

**Step 3:** Grab the lower mass of hair and tie it back with a hair tie. (Don't worry—this won't be seen once you are done.)

**Step 4:** Untie the top section and work your pomade, styling gel, or mousse into it.

**Step 5:** Grab your bobby pins, pull that top section back, and pin it to the back of your head as securely as possible to prevent the hair from flopping about. (I know it looks messy but trust me, we got this!)

**Step 6:** Take a hair scarf and fold it in half. Place the largest part of the scarf on the back of your hair, making sure it covers your rubber band and bobby pins.

**Step 7:** Now give your scarf a good tug.

**Step 8:** Tie it in a beautiful bow, and there you have it!

**Step 9:** For extra precaution to ensure our scarf doesn't slip, grab a couple of bobby pins and pin your scarf to your hair on both sides.

**You're set:** Boom, baby! Go out into the world and pinup-slay!

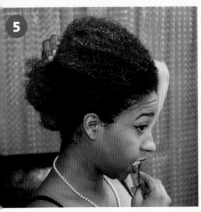

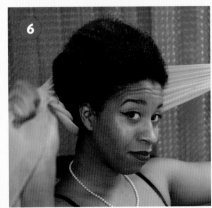

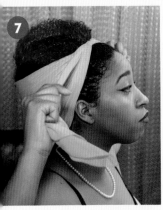

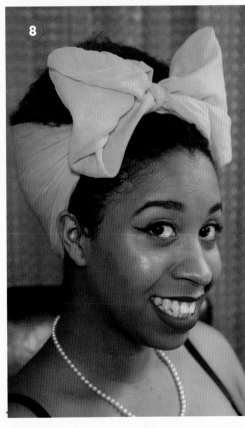

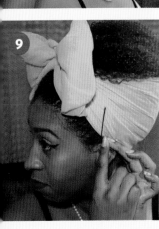

# PINUP MAKEUP

The good news for the less beauty-savvy among us is that pinup makeup is generally much simpler than today's often intimidating techniques. The basic face of classic '50s pinup is always a sure bet and easy to achieve. In fact, it's likely you can do most of what you usually do and then add a cat eye (also referred to as winged eyeliner).

Lots of pinups find it most convenient to do their makeup while their curls set. Starting with clean, moisturized skin, apply sunscreen (if not in your moisturizer), face primer, foundation, and concealer. Set with powder, and then sweep on some blush (try a pink, coral, or reddish shade). Define your brows with a gel, pencil, or powder in a shade slightly darker than your natural tint to make them stand out a bit and frame the cat eye you'll do next (mascara and lipstick to follow). You probably know or will soon discover if you prefer to do these steps in a different order. Do what works best for you!

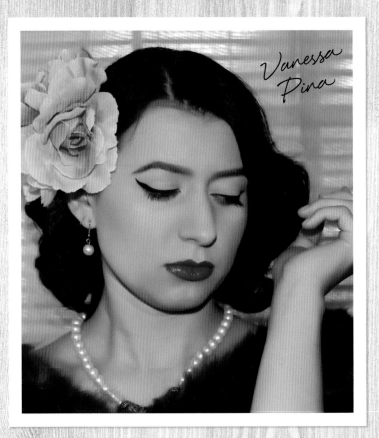

Vanessa
Pina

# Winged Eyeliner How To

**STYLIST AND PHOTOGRAPHER:** Lyla Blush
**MODEL:** Vanessa Pina

# supplies needed

Experiment with the various types of eyeliner to see which one works best for you. For this look, options include brush-tip or felt-tip liquid liner, or a gel liner pot with a slim brush. In addition, you can use a nude, flesh-toned pencil eyeliner on the lower waterline.

Make sure you have applied your favorite eye primer, base foundation, or concealer to the eye area before starting your eyeliner.

# how to

**Step 1:** Start with clean skin. Be sure to apply your primer product, whichever is your favorite to use, then apply eye shadow (typically something neutral for a classic look—taupe is always a safe bet).

**Step 2:** Looking straight ahead into the mirror, relax your face, and, using a liquid liner or gel, draw the outline of where you want your wing to be. Begin from your lower lash line and aim toward the end of your brow, then in toward your lid, making the wing as thick or as thin as you prefer.

**Step 3:** Continue to draw your line, narrowing toward the inside edge of your iris. You want to line all the way to the tear duct, but keep the line on the inside of your eye minimal and thin.

**Step 4:** Fill in the area drawn with your eyeliner. The illusion is that the liner appears to be straight when the eye is open, but actually it's not as you can see in the sample photo. (This model has hooded eyes, which many women find difficult to do winged eyeliner on. If you do not have hooded eyes, the line would be curved down onto the lid when closed.)

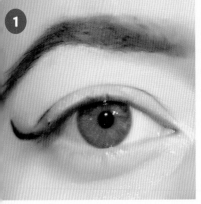

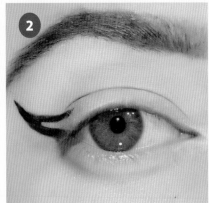

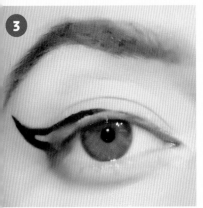

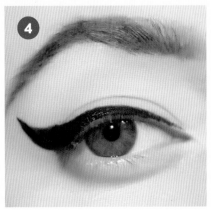

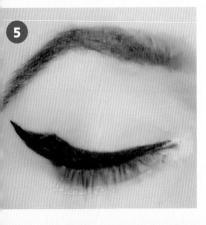

**Step 5:** Line the lower waterline with the nude, flesh-toned liner, and add mascara to the lashes. Add false lashes if you want more drama.

Top off the look with your favorite shade of red lip liner and lipstick.

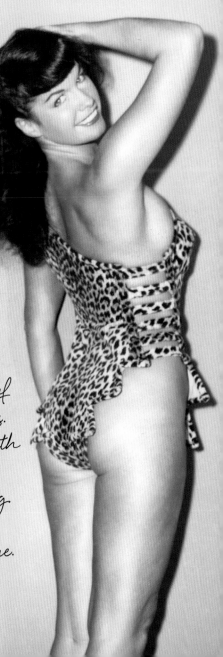

## CHAPTER SIX

# THE BEAUTY, PART II:

# PINUP STYLE

*They claim that I'm an instigator of a lot of the styles. I never kept up with the fashions. I believed in wearing what I thought looked good on me.*

*—Bettie Page*

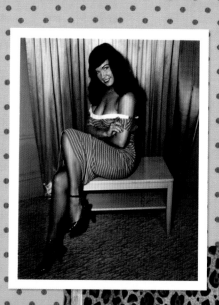
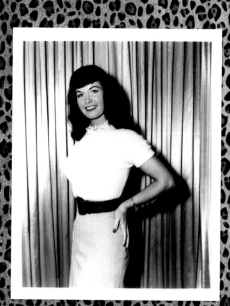

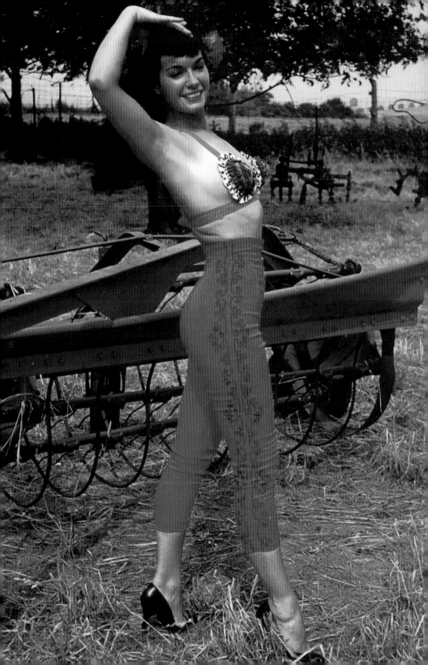

*B*ETTIE KNEW EXACTLY HOW SHE WANTED her clothes to fit her, and it usually wasn't like the ones she found in stores or catalogs. So she often hand-made her own, especially the bikinis she wore in photo shoots and at a time when wearing any bikini in public was taboo, it's highly unlikely she would have found the kind she wanted if she hadn't made them herself.

Like their creator, Bettie's styles were distinctive and innovative—so good that a clothing company she modeled for copied her designs and hawked them as their own, using her name and photos. When she wasn't modeling, her public outfits were usually stylish but simple: a blouse and capris, a no-frills dress, or a pencil skirt and sweater with minimal jewelry. (She did, however, vamp it up privately; there are a number of gorgeous photos of her posing nude and in lingerie for a man she dated named Charles West.) Of course, that was just Bettie's preference, and the best way to honor her is to wear what makes *you* feel best, whether understated, over-the-top, or somewhere in between.

This guide will help you begin exploring your personal pinup style.

OPPOSITE: High-waisted pants paired with another of Bettie's handmade bikini tops. PREVIOUS SPREAD: Bettie's DIY swimsuit and other Bettie fashions

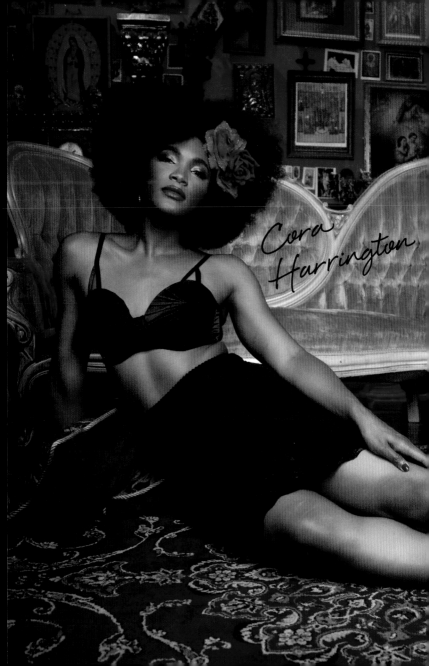

Cora Harrington

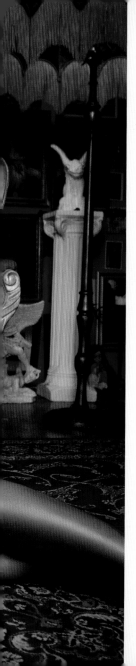

# PINUP LINGERIE 101

This section is by Cora Harrington, founder and editor-in-chief of The Lingerie Addict (Thelingerieaddict.com) and author of *In Intimate Detail: How to Choose, Wear, and Love Lingerie.*

Who is possibly a more iconic pinup than Bettie Page? While her hairstyle, her poses, and even her shoes are known the world over, what I love most about Bettie is her lingerie. From diaphanous tulle gowns to figure-hugging corsets to scandalously skimpy bralettes, the lingerie Bettie Page wore managed to be both timeless and modern, vintage yet of the moment. Her captivating ensembles help to explain why, even decades later, we still can't get enough of her photographs. Ready to put together your own Bettie Page—inspired lingerie drawer? Here's what you need to know.

# The Essentials

The classic pinup shape is the dramatic hourglass figure with a high, uplifted (some might even say "pointy") bosom and a cinched-in waist. Vintage-inspired underpinnings are necessary to achieve this silhouette. Here are the basics:

**Bullet Bra:** Known for their "torpedo" cups and circular stitching, bullet bras are indispensable for a 1950s-style figure. If you can't find a bullet bra, look for a seamed or "fully-fashioned" bra. These bras are readily identifiable by a pronounced seam across the middle of the bust as well as a seam running from the bottom of the cup to the middle. While old-fashioned looking, those seams are what create that vintage shape.

**High-Waisted Briefs or Tap Pants:** Thongs existed in the 1950s (mostly on the burlesque circuit), but they weren't considered mainstream just yet. For that authentic vintage lingerie model silhouette, you want a full-coverage knicker. Look for styles made from satin or lace for the ultimate retro look. As an added bonus, these fabrics help to avoid panty lines under your pencil skirts!

**Girdle or Waist Cincher:** Vintage-style shapewear supports and smooths the body, giving a toned, "tight" look under clothing. Girdles can be of the open-bottom variety (a bit like a very short skirt) or a closed–bottom–panty girdle style. Girdles can also end right at the waist, where they focus on shaping the hips and rear, or extend as far as the bra band, sculpting the waist and torso as well (this is

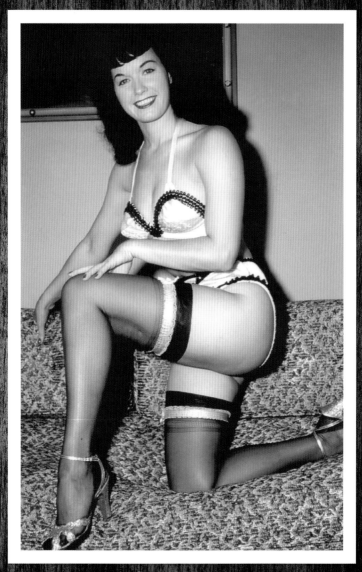

Bettie's DIY lingerie

called a "longline" girdle). Girdles with a built-in bra are called corselettes or body briefers. Shapewear that focuses exclusively on nipping in the waist is called a waist cincher.

**Garter Belts:** They are amazingly versatile and one of the most provocative kinds of lingerie ever invented. A high-quality garter belt, the type someone would have worn daily in the 1950s, has a minimum of six garter straps: two at the front, two at the sides, and two at the back. All those garters help to keep your stockings from twisting, falling down, or tearing. Garter belts are worn at the natural waist. The natural flare of your hipbones will help keep your suspenders in place.

**Stockings:** A true, Bettie Page–era stocking is made from 100 percent nylon and is either fully-fashioned (with a back seam and keyhole welt) or RHT (a reinforced heel and toe). Stockings that are 100 percent nylon have no stretch and are incredibly delicate. Therefore, you'll want to pay close attention to the size chart before purchasing. For all their trouble, the way they look on the leg is worth it!

**Slip:** No vintage lingerie collection is complete without a slip. While slips are worn underneath skirts and dresses to help them drape better as well as to protect your outerwear from sweat or oil, they're also unbelievably glamorous in their own right and make for perfect lounging attire. Buy a satin slip (made from either nylon or silk) for maximum versatility.

**Dressing Gowns:** Round out your lingerie wardrobe with a voluminous, over-the-top dressing gown. Dressing gowns are like the dramatic big sister to robes. Ideally, they're floor-length with huge sleeves, perfect for wearing in front of the mirror while you perfect your Bettie Page pout!

# Where to Buy

Now that you know the essentials and can call yourself a Bettie Page lingerie expert, here are a few places to shop!

Bettiepagelingerie.com (of course!)

Whatkatiedid.com

Dottiesdelights.com

Rago-shapewear.com

Kissmedeadly.co.uk

Cocosretrocloset.com

Goddessbra.com

Stockingshq.com

Secretsinlace.com

Boudoirbydlish.com

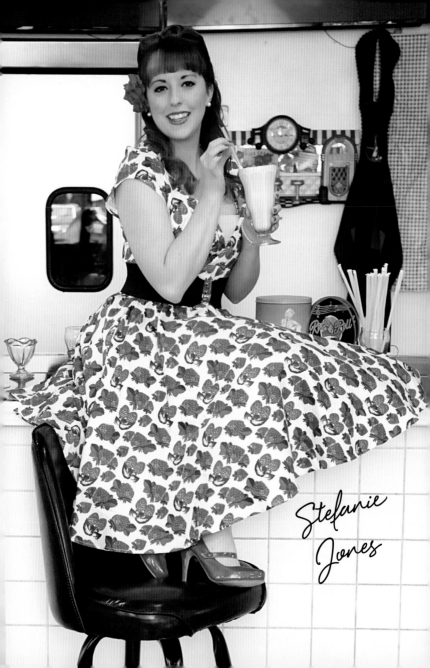

Stefanie
Jones

# PINUP CLOTHING 101

This section is by Stefanie Jones, owner of Junk Drunk Jones (Junkdrunkjones.com), an antiques store in Canton, Georgia, that boasts a large collection of vintage and vintage-inspired clothing and accessories.

The pinup style guarantees a level of uniqueness that not many styles can boast and it lends a lot of creativity. There isn't a magical formula that everyone must follow, so I will make some suggestions, and the rest is up to you! To create outfits that combine perfectly with pinup-style hair and makeup, score the staples below. And don't be afraid to pair a few vintage-style items with your everyday clothes for some fun flair. We don't have to be 100 percent pinup all day, every day, but you will be surprised at the compliments and attention you will receive when you start incorporating elements of this look into your life.

# Building the Wardrobe

**Dresses:** Start with three or four dresses to cover you for special events, parties, and potential photo shoots. There are typically two primary styles when it comes to the 1950s: swing dresses lend more "room" for moving around and can be worn with a petticoat underneath (optional), while wiggle dresses are form-fitting, typically knee-length, and show all your curves (very Bettie indeed!). Once you scoop up a few dresses and wear them while you're out and about, you will be able to tweak your personal preferences.

**Skirts:** Start with two or three skirts. Again, there are two primary styles for this era: Swing skirts are like the dresses, but give you more options because you can pair them with various tops. Then there are the form-fitting pencil skirts. For both, the prints and fabric options are plentiful, so you can decide how wild or tame you want to be.

**Bottoms:** You probably already have a certain staple in your closet: skinny jeans! Cuff them at the bottom, and boom, you are ready! These can be dressed up or down: Pair with a cute top and heels to go bombshell, or add a tee and some flats for a comfy look. You may also want to snag some high-waisted shorts, so keep an eye out for these as you shop.

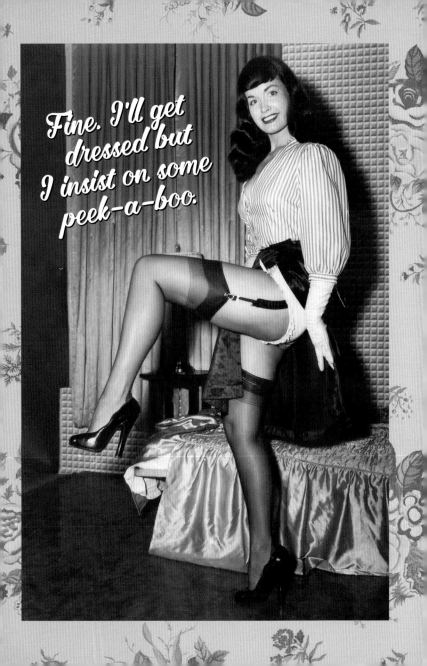

Fine. I'll get dressed but I insist on some peek-a-boo.

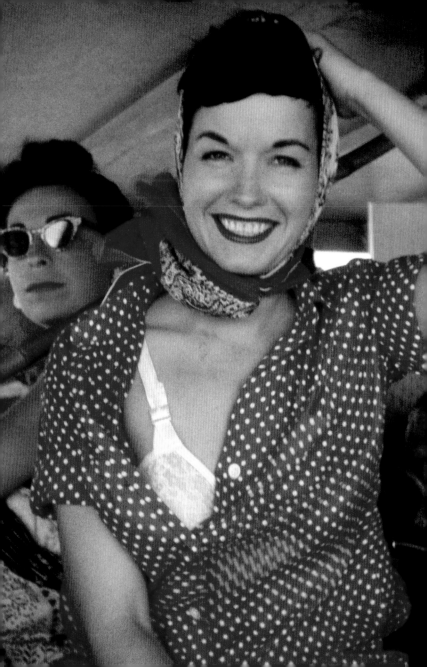

**Shoes:** A few pairs each of heels and flats should do the trick. The heels: What do you typically wear already? Whether you are a wedge or stiletto type of gal doesn't matter—they both complement the pinup look well. I would recommend a solid black heel and a solid red heel as those pair very well with the patterns found in vintage and vintage-inspired clothing items. For the flats, a nice pair of converse "Chucks" or saddle oxfords are a great start.

**Tops:** I recommend three or four tops to pair with the skirts and bottoms. Solid-colored blouses are key, but that really depends on how wild you got with the prints of your skirts and such. I am no stranger to matching stripes with leopard print, so if you are as quirky as I am, go right ahead with the loud prints! Cardigans are a godsend for the vintage look—a few can make your wardrobe. Button the top button, or use some cute sweater clips to hold the top of your cardigan together.

**Accessories:** Starting a collection of unique costume jewelry items can be so much fun! The '50s gals loved their brooches, flowers, cute animals, and sparkly baubles. A set of pearl earrings are always a nice touch. There are lots of vintage and vintage-inspired handbag options. Cat eye–shaped sunglasses are a cool addition, and be sure to buy some bandannas or hair scarves for your pinup updos.

## 10 STYLE LESSONS FROM
# Bettie Page

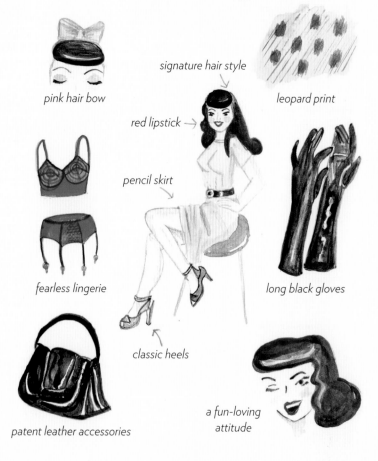

pink hair bow

signature hair style

leopard print

red lipstick →

pencil skirt

fearless lingerie

long black gloves

patent leather accessories

classic heels

a fun-loving attitude

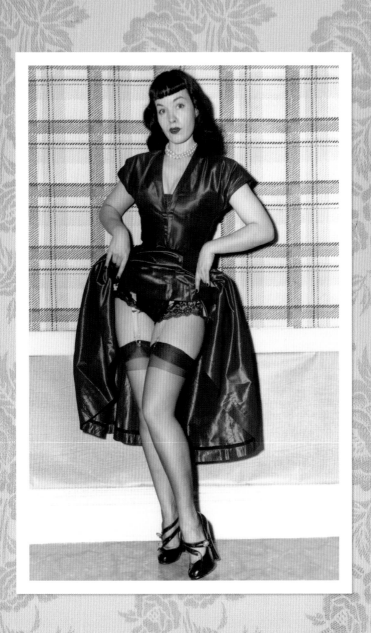

# Shopping for the Wardrobe

Clearly, the most entertaining part of achieving this look is shopping for it. You might find what you're looking for at these places:

**Thrift Stores:** This is probably the more time-consuming suggestion, but could also provide a gold mine for you. If you are not opposed to doing some digging to score a few pieces, then check out your local thrift shops for the chance to acquire some authentic vintage items.

**Etsy:** This is a great online resource because the items are primarily handmade or vintage, and the site is super-searchable. Insider tip: If you are browsing a specific Etsy shop and you just love several pieces, send them a polite message telling them so, and ask if they would be willing to offer a discount for the entire lot.

**Retailers:** A wonderful way to shop for vintage and vintage-inspired items is through brick-and-mortar shops like mine. We are on hand to help with questions or specific needs, and we have dressing areas to eliminate guesswork. Search for boutiques and antiques stores in your area that stock pinup-style clothing, shoes, and accessories.

# Where to Buy

For online shopping, solid options include:

| | |
|---|---|
| Bettiepage.com | Modcloth.com |
| Heartofhaute.com | Voodoovixen.co.uk |
| Pinupgirlclothing.com | Zoevine.com |
| Retroglam.com | Joanieclothing.com |
| Unique-vintage.com | Hellbunny.com |
| Dollmeupdarling.com | Stopstaringclothing.com |
| Collectif.co.uk | Heydayonline.co.uk |
| Lindybopusa.com | Baitfootwear.com |
| Topvintage.net/en | Chaseandchloe.com |
| Theprettydresscompany.com | Chelseacrew.com |
| Trashydiva.com | |

Be wary about sizing when buying true vintage clothing online, as it is very different from modern sizing. Pay attention to actual garment measurements, and ask for specifics if you aren't sure. Returns can be a hassle with private sellers, so do your homework before ordering.

Have fun creating your pinup wardrobe, and remember: You are beautiful, and you look amazing!

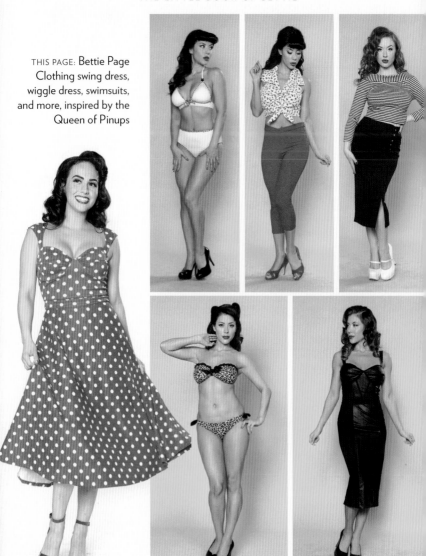

THIS PAGE: **Bettie Page** Clothing swing dress, wiggle dress, swimsuits, and more, inspired by the Queen of Pinups

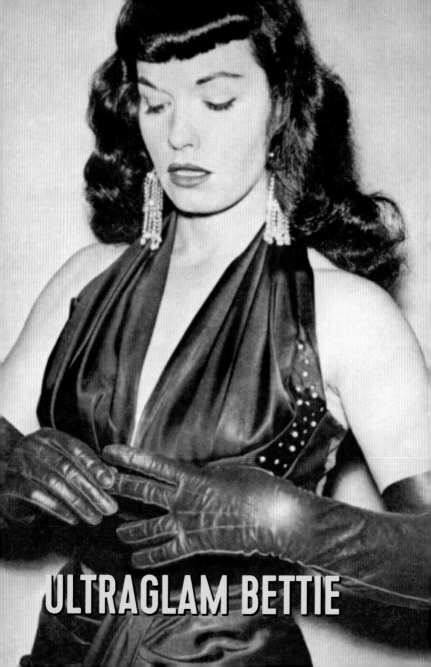

ULTRAGLAM BETTIE

# Pinup for All!

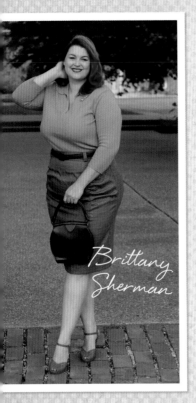

*Brittany Sherman*

I believe that pinup style is for everyone. I'm a mom of two and I often volunteer at my kids' school, teaching crafts at the class parties and chaperoning events. For those occasions, I stick to the basics with a great-fitting-knee-length pencil skirt, easy wash-and-wear knit top, and a quick hot roller set. I love my vintage-style heels, but I usually keep a pair of black flats in my purse for chasing the kids at the park after school.

—BRITTANY SHERMAN,
blogger at Vavoom Vintage
(Vavoomvintage.net)

Bettie Page is not only the "Queen of Pinups," but perhaps the queen of budget-conscious chic, with her DIY outfits. There's a common misconception that pinup fashion requires an extravagant wallet—not so. I've put together looks for under $50. One thrifty tip: For a busy pinup, nylon and chiffon scarves are practically essential. Make a quick DIY scarf by cutting a 23 x 23-inch square out of nylon fabric from your local fabric store.

—MISS VELVET WREN,
administrator of Pinups of Colour

# CHAPTER SEVEN
## the BRAINS

I used to make most
of my clothes, at least
half of them—my dresses,
blouses, and skirts. I had
fun designing those bikinis.
They were an outrage then
in America. Only over
in France and other
places in Europe
were they worn.

—Bettie Page

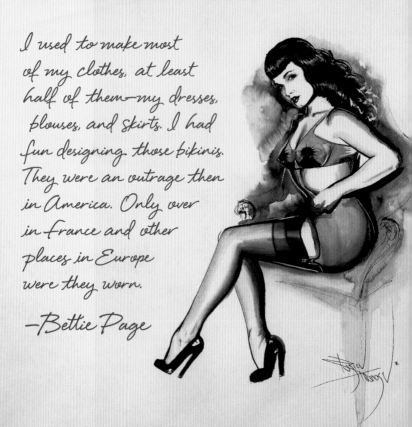

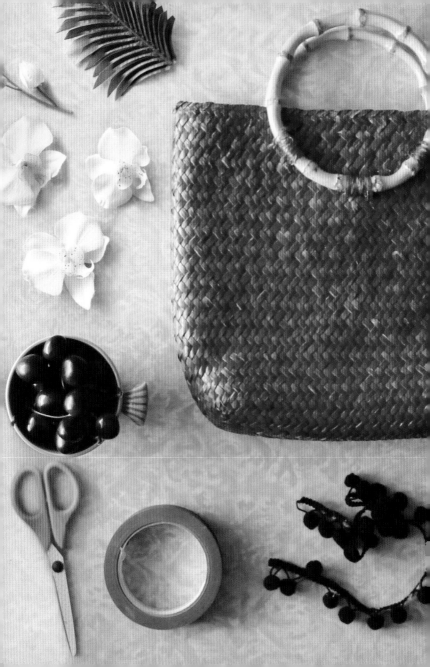

*O*F THE COUNTLESS COOL THINGS ABOUT BETTIE, her remarkable creativity and curiosity are key features. Along with all her DIY designs and modeling genius, she loved to explore and learn new things, and she frequently studied arts, like music and acting. Her influence has helped to nurture the creative pursuits of her fans, too, and she often serves as the muse herself. Women regularly recreate her image and poses for photo shoots, and burlesque performers draw inspiration from her attitude and playful moves. For Thèrese Rosier, an artist from Prague, Bettie boosted her self-confidence back in her school days and later became a frequent subject of her art. "As a painter, she's been my inspiration for the last fifteen years, since art school. She is just the perfect 'object' to paint, and it is always a pleasure to do it."

If you've been wanting to tap your creative side (and you do have one, I promise) or see what this DIY stuff is all about, try one or all of these totally unintimidating pinup-perfect craft projects, inspired by Bettie and created just for you by Brittany Sherman of Vavoom Vintage (Vavoomvintage.net).

PREVIOUS SPREAD: Bettie Page painting by Thérèse Rosier

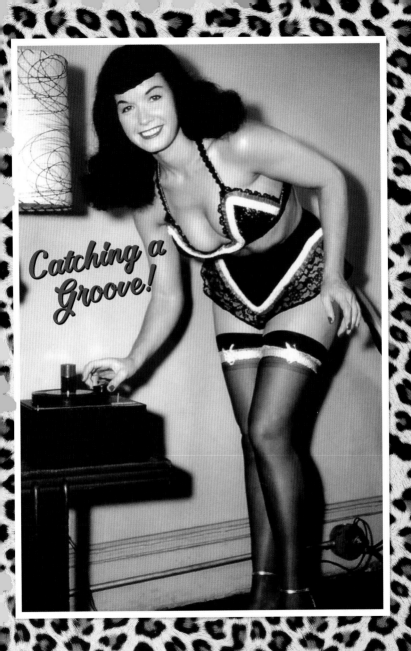

Catching a Groove!

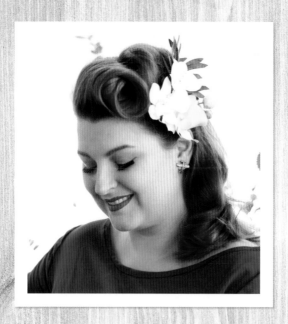

# TROPICAL HAIR FLOWER

Hair flowers were popular accessories throughout the 1940s and '50s. Wear them with elaborate victory rolls or elegant pageboy hairstyles. Here's how to make your own collection of hair flowers for any occasion. Faux flowers come in a range of quality. You can find very inexpensive ones at the dollar store or on sale at local craft stores. Some higher-end flowers are made of foam or rubber and look just like the real thing! For this project, I'm using orchids in white and orange and some tropical greenery.

## supplies needed

- ○ Scissors or wire cutters
- ○ Faux flowers of your choice
- ○ Hot glue gun and sticks
- ○ Craft felt of your color choice
- ○ Hair clip

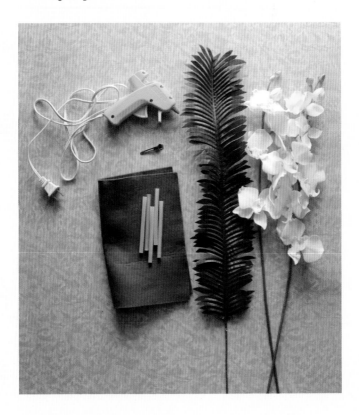

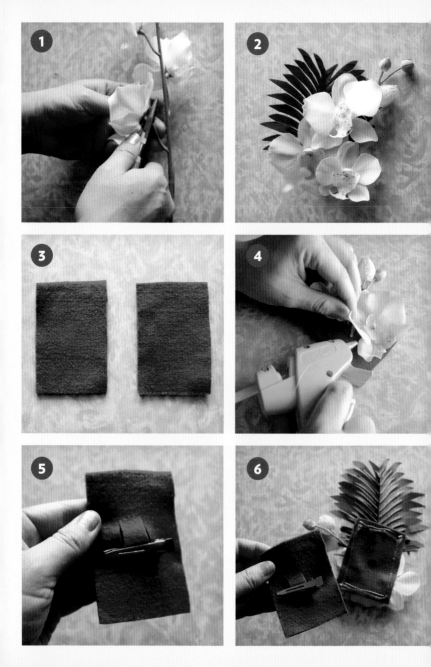

# *how to*

**Step 1:** Cut the flowers from the stem. Sometimes the flowers will come apart when they are no longer attached to the stem. If they do, a little dot of hot glue will hold the petals together.

**Step 2:** Arrange your flowers to your liking. I like to cluster an odd number of smaller flowers around a central focal point, or if the flowers are all the same size, alternate colors asymmetrically. Add the dramatic flourishes of greenery or a sprig of flower buds in the back.

**Step 3:** Cut two pieces of felt for the base of your flower. The size and shape may differ, depending on what flowers you're using. I cut 2 rectangles about 3 x 2 inches.

**Step 4:** Glue your flowers to one of the felt bases. You can glue edges of petals and leaves to each other to hold the arrangement in place securely.

**Step 5:** On the other base, cut two small parallel slits for the hair clip to slide into.

**Step 6:** Glue the two bases together around the outer edges.

Use these steps to make a collection of hair flowers for every occasion. Find small wreath picks with little retro starburst shapes around the holidays, or go spooky with spiders, pumpkins, and little skeleton parts for Halloween. Add small plastic fruit and gingham bows for summer or crisp white feathers, flowers, and beads for a bridal look.

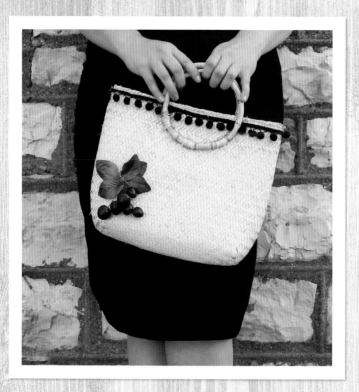

# PINUP-STYLE STRAW PURSE

A fabulous handbag adds instant pinup style to any outfit.
This project turns a basic thrift-store purse into a kitschy
one-of-a-kind handbag with an ode to Bettie in the no-sew
animal print lining.

# *supplies needed*

- ○ **Pom-pom trim**
- ○ **Faux cherries and a few leaves**
- ○ **Scrap of craft felt**
- ○ **Hot glue gun and glue sticks**
- ○ **Straw or wicker purse**
- ○ **Spray paint in your choice of color and painter's tape (optional)**

## Supplies Needed for No-Sew Lining (Optional)

- ○ 1/2 yard fabric
- ○ Iron-on adhesive, such as Heat 'n Bond or Stitch Witchery
- ○ Tape measure
- ○ Iron

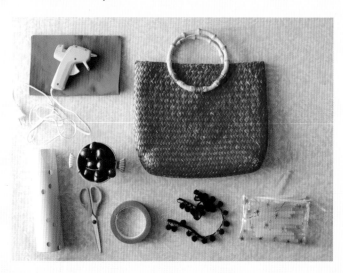

# *how to*

**Step 1:** Look for a straw purse with good bones at the thrift store. Make sure the straw is strong and the handles are sturdy. If you would like to paint your purse, mask off the handles and hardware with painter's tape and take it to a well-ventilated area or outside. Spray several light, even coats, allowing it to dry between coats. When one side looks good, flip it over and repeat, being sure to paint the bottom as well.

**Step 2:** Measure a length of pom-pom trim to fit along the top opening of your purse. Cut to size and hot-glue it into place, gluing just a few inches at a time.

**Step 3:** Cut a small 2-inch circle of craft felt. Glue the cherries by the stems to the circle of felt. Add a few leaves to cover the felt.

**Step 4:** Glue the sprig of cherries to your bag.

**Step 5:** For the no-sew lining, measure your bag and make note of the height and width. Cut two pieces of fabric 1 inch larger (in width and height) than the bag. If your bag is box-shaped, you will also need to cut pieces for the sides and bottom of the purse and iron them together to form a box, as explained below.

**Step 6:** With the right side up, lay a strip of iron-on adhesive along the bottom edge of the fabric.

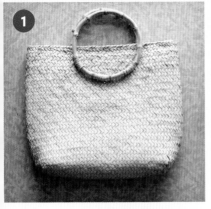

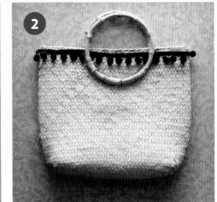

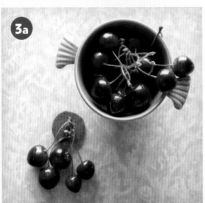

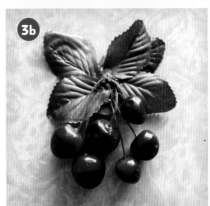

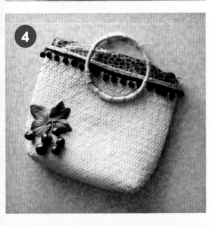

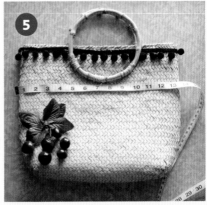

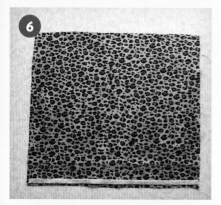

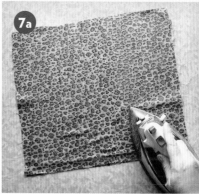

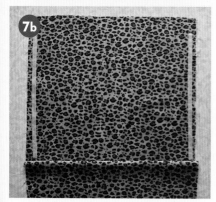

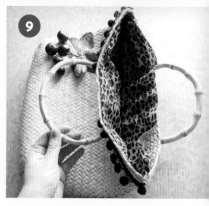

**Step 7:** Lay the other piece of fabric on top (right side down) and iron them together. Repeat on both sides. Check the seams to make sure they have bonded together.

**Step 8:** Insert the lining into the purse and press the seam edges along the seams of the purse so everything fits nicely.

**Step 9:** Fold the top opening of the lining down about a half inch and glue the lining to the purse along the top opening.

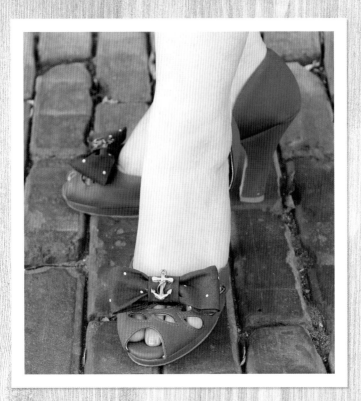

# NAUTICAL SHOE CLIPS

Dress up your favorite sky-high heels or practical flats with these nautical no-sew shoe clips. Change up the fabric print and themed charms to craft a collection of easy accessories that you can wear anywhere!

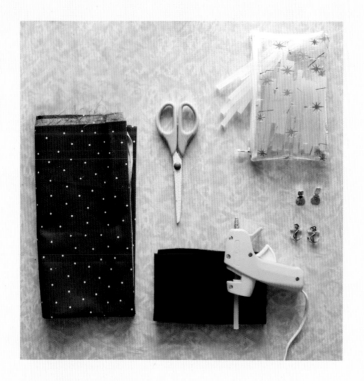

## supplies needed

- ○ Pair of shoe clips
- ○ Scissors
- ○ Fabric remnant (I'm using a cute navy polka-dot cotton)
- ○ Hot glue gun and glue sticks
- ○ Scrap of craft felt
- ○ Pair of nautical charms

## prep steps

Cut 2 rectangles 8 x 6 inches.

Cut 2 rectangles 3 x 2 inches.

Cut 2 small circles out of
the felt.

## how to for
## each clip

**Step 1:** Fold one of the larger
rectangles into thirds with
the right side out so the raw
edges meet in the middle. Fold
lengthwise once more.

**Step 2:** Fold the edges over to
meet in the middle and glue
into place.

**Step 3:** Pinch in the middle to
make a bow shape. Glue the
middle to hold the bow shape.

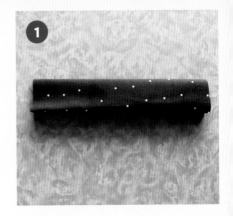

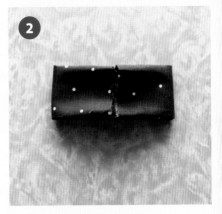

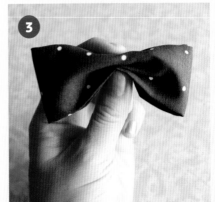

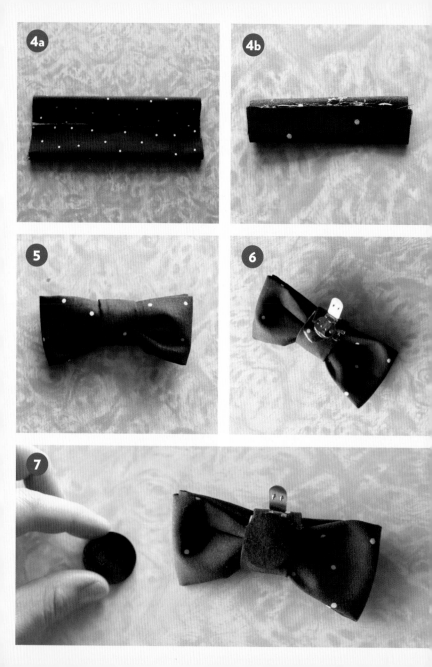

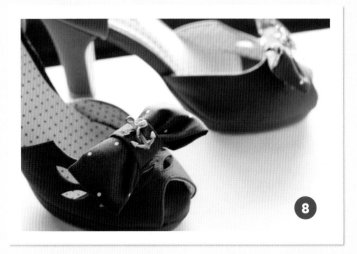

**Step 4:** Fold one of the smaller rectangles into thirds lengthwise and glue it into place so the raw edge is on the back.

**Step 5:** Wrap around the middle of the bow and glue it into place.

**Step 6:** Open your shoe clip and glue it to the back of the bow.

**Step 7:** Glue the dots of felt to the back of the shoe clip.

**Step 8:** Glue or sew your nautical charms to the front of the bow, as shown above.

# How to Pick a Pinup Name

## by MISS TAYLOR NICOLE

If you're considering joining the pinup community, you're probably toying with the idea of adopting a pinup name. By no means do you need to have one, but they are fun to create and can help give you recognition on the vintage scene. Here are a few simple tips to help you find a wonderful and unique name.

TIP 1: Get inspired. This may seem obvious, but a lot of pinups get stuck at this point. It can be as simple as looking up your favorite pinup models and considering what you like about their name: Does it have wordplay (like Ursula Undress's take on Ursula Andress)? Did they reference something? Is it alliterative? Once you figure out what stood out to you about their name, try to include that same type of concept in your pinup name.

TIP 2: Make it about you. Inspiration is great, but you don't want to copy another pinup's name. If you make it distinctive, then it will be easy to come up with something new. You can use your grandmother's name, your favorite color, or even your favorite location.

TIP 3: Stick with it. Once you've chosen a pinup name, you don't want to change it every month. Even though it may not be set in stone, if you change it too often you risk being forgotten or losing your following. Of course, if you suddenly decide that you hate the name you picked, change it! Just be mindful, especially if you've already built up a following.

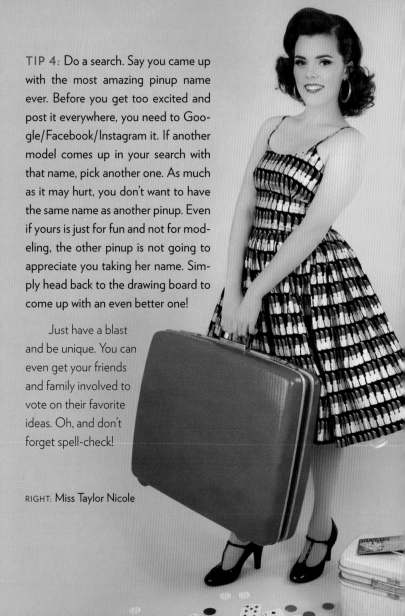

TIP 4: Do a search. Say you came up with the most amazing pinup name ever. Before you get too excited and post it everywhere, you need to Google/Facebook/Instagram it. If another model comes up in your search with that name, pick another one. As much as it may hurt, you don't want to have the same name as another pinup. Even if yours is just for fun and not for modeling, the other pinup is not going to appreciate you taking her name. Simply head back to the drawing board to come up with an even better one!

Just have a blast and be unique. You can even get your friends and family involved to vote on their favorite ideas. Oh, and don't forget spell-check!

RIGHT: Miss Taylor Nicole

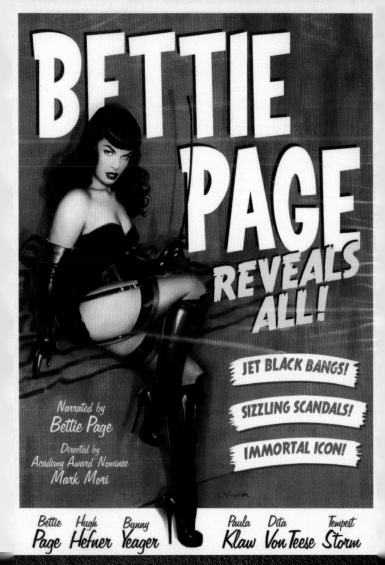

# THE BRAND

Since CMG Worldwide started managing the use of Bettie's image after the connection was made through Hugh Hefner, the Bettie Page brand has become a multimillion-dollar enterprise with substantial growth each year. Businesses that are interested in licensing Bettie's image are carefully screened to ensure that her legacy is respected and preserved. Check out this sampling of Bettie businesses.

**Bettie Page Clothing:** The main attraction on the official Bettie Page website offers tons of fun, colorful, Bettie-inspired dresses, swimsuits, and separates that are made in the USA by Coral & Jade Apparel.

**Olivia de Berardinis:** She has been famously making impeccable paintings of Bettie for many years, and she designed the cover art for the *Bettie Page Reveals All* documentary. She sells prints and other merchandise—including rolling papers—featuring her Bettie art.

**Bettie Page Shoes by Ellie Shoes:** These are a favorite on the pinup scene. The collection "caters to the lifestyle and inspirations of Bettie Page's iconic presence within the subcultures that follow her today," according to their website.

BELOW: Shoes by Bettie Page Shoes

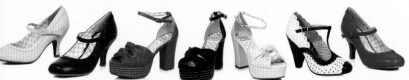

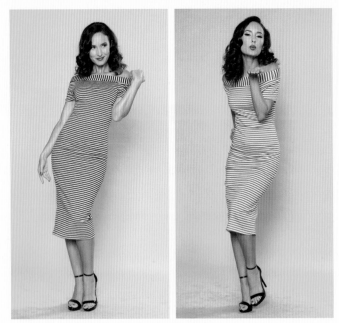

ABOVE: Bettie Page Clothing by Coral & Jade

**Bettie Page Lingerie:** Launched by Playful Promises, a UK-based intimates company that carries a wide range of sizes, the line embraces body positivity and fights ageism and racism through its ad campaigns.

**Dynamite Comics:** A new comic book series starring Bettie was launched by Dynamite in 2017.

**Bettie Page Wine and Bettie Page Rum:** They are produced by the California-based Sort This Out Cellars, which also serves the rum at its very own tiki bar. Each new edition of the wine features a different Bettie-centric label.

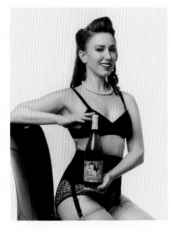
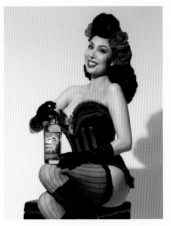

ABOVE PHOTOS BY RADIANT INC. FROM LEFT: **Bettie Page Wine** modeled by Millie Michelle; **Bettie Page Rum** modeled by Kalani Kokonuts. BELOW: handbags by Bettie Page Handbags

**Bettie Page Handbags by Lola Ramona:** These are cute retro-style bags made with Bettie in mind—some even featuring the silhouette of her face from one of her photos.

**Retro-a-go-go!:** A Michigan-based online store that sells tons of original accessories and novelty items bearing Bettie's image, including parasols, signs, flasks, cigarette cases, and more.

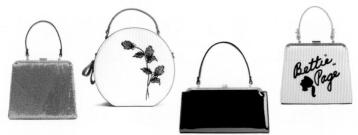

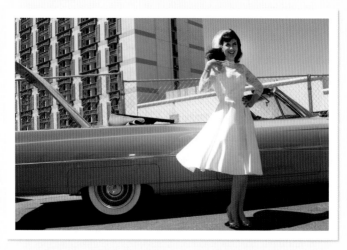

ABOVE: Pinup model Lilla Rosten wearing her Bettie Page wedding dress by Bettie Page Bridal. Her wedding was sponsored by Bettie Page brands and took place at the Viva Las Vegas Rockabilly Weekender.

**Bettie Bangs:** A clip-in version of the classic 'do that is made from 100 percent human hair by California-based Classy Rebel. They also make Bettie Page wigs!

**Bettie Page Bridal & Formal by Heart of Haute:** They make vintage-style Bettie-inspired wedding dresses, bridesmaids dresses, and more. Lilla Rosten, a pinup model from Australia, won a Bettie Page wedding that was held at the Viva Las Vegas Rockabilly Weekender in 2016. It was sponsored by CMG and all the Bettie licensees, including Bettie Page Bridal, which donated the dress to the bride.

**Bettie Page Fitness:** My own line produces body-positive workout videos that are fully inspired by the Queen of Pinups, and designed and taught by me!

# BIBLIOGRAPHY

## INTRODUCTION

Sharkey, Lorelei. "Not the Pin-Up We Played Her For: An Interview with Bettie Page." Nerve.com, 1998. http://www.nerve.com/dispatches/page/pinuplegend, accessed July 31, 2017.

## CHAPTER ONE:
## THE BETTIE BABES

Goldsmith, Jeffrey. "Bettie Page Interview." *Make You Famous*, November 4, 2016. http://makeyoufamous.co/bettie-page-interview, accessed July 31, 2017.

"Katy Perry and Madonna on the Power of Pop." *V* magazine, summer 2014, issue 89.

Hirschberg, Lynn. "Beyoncé Talks Fashion: The artist comments on the seven looks that shaped her career. *W* magazine, July 1, 2010. https://www.wmagazine.com/gallery/beyonce-video-looks-ss/all, accessed July 31, 2017.

"Archetype." Dictionary.com. http://www.dictionary.com/browse/archetype, accessed July 31, 2017.

## CHAPTER TWO:
## THE BACKSTORY

Sharkey, Lorelei. "Not the Pin-Up We Played Her For: An Interview with Bettie Page." Nerve.com, 1998. http://www.nerve.com/dispatches/page/pinuplegend, accessed July 31, 2017.

"About Bettie Page: Biography." https://www.bettiepage.com/about, accessed July 31, 2017.

"Bettie Page Visits the Mr. Showbiz Celebrity Lounge." *Mr. Showbiz Celebrity Lounge*. March 1996. http://www.grrl.com/chat.html, accessed July 31, 2017.

Carlson, Michael. "Bettie Page." *The Guardian,* December 12, 2008. https://www.theguardian.com/film/2008/dec/13/obituary-bettie-page, accessed July 31, 2017.

*Bettie Page Reveals All*. Directed by Mark Mori. 2013. Chicago, IL: Music Box Films, 2013. DVD/Blu-ray

Bass, Mary Tom. "Bettie Page: The Pinup of Peabody." *Peabody Reflector,* winter 2003. https://www.vanderbilt.edu/wp-content/uploads/sites/90/archives/2003-Winter-Peabody-Reflector.pdf, accessed July 31, 2017.

"Percentage of the U.S. Population Who Have Completed Four Years of College or More from 1940 to 2016, By Gender." *Statista*. https://www.statista.com/statistics/184272/educational-attainment-of-college-diploma-or-higher-by-gender, accessed July 31, 2017.

"Bettie Page Dies." *ComicMix*, December 12, 2008. http://www.comicmix.com/2008/12/12/bettie-page-dies, accessed July 31, 2017.

"About Bettie Page: Quotes." www.bettiepage.com/quotes, accessed July 31, 2017.

Rodriguez, Tori. "Male Fans Made Bettie Page a Star, but Female Fans Made Her an Icon." *The Atlantic,* January 6, 2014. https://www.theatlantic.com/entertainment/archive/2014/01/male-fans-made-bettie-page-a-star-but-female-fans-made-her-an-icon/282794, accessed July 31, 2017.

"Bettie Page Talks God, Love and Bondage." *American Suburb X,* June 10, 2015 (transcribed from September 1998 interview). http://www.americansuburbx.com/2015/06/interview-interview-with-bettie-page-1998.html, accessed July 31, 2017.

Cook, Kevin. "Bettie Page: The Missing Years." *Playboy,* January 1998. http://atlantisonline.smfforfree2.com/index.php?topic=3944.0;wap2, accessed July 31, 2017.

Perrone, Pierre. "Bettie Page: Queen of the Fifties pin-ups who became a cult figure." *The Independent,* December 13, 2008. http://www.independent.co.uk/news/obituaries/bettie-page-queen-of-the-fifties-pin-ups-who-became-a-cult-figure-1064499.html, accessed July 31, 2017.

"1950s Pinup Model Bettie Page Dead at 85." CNN, December 12, 2008. http://www.cnn.com/2008/US/12/12/bettie.page.obit, accessed July 31, 2017.

O'Malley-Greenburg, Zack. "The Highest-Paid Dead Celebrities of 2016." *Forbes,* October 12, 2016. https://www.forbes.com/sites/zackomalleygreenburg/2016/10/12/the-highest-paid-dead-celebrities-of-2016/#39b32d0311b1, accessed July 31, 2017.

Grow, Kory. "See John Lydon Praise Bettie Page in New Public Image Ltd. Video." *Rolling Stone,* October 29, 2015. http://www.rollingstone.com/music/news/see-john-lydon-praise-bettie-page-in-new-public-image-ltd-video-20151029, accessed July 31, 2017.

CHAPTER THREE:
**THE BOLDNESS**

Goldsmith, Jeffrey. "Bettie Page Interview." *Make You Famous,* November 4, 2016. http://makeyoufamous.co/bettie-page-interview, accessed July 31, 2017.

"Bettie Page Talks God, Love and Bondage." *American Suburb X,* June 10, 2015 (transcribed from September 1998 interview). http://www.americansuburbx.com/2015/06/interview-interview-with-bettie-page-1998.html, accessed July 31, 2017

Sharkey, Lorelei. "Not the Pin-Up We Played Her For: An Interview with Bettie Page." Nerve.com, 1998. http://www.nerve.com/dispatches/page/pinuplegend, accessed July 31, 2017.

Rodriguez, Tori. "Here's What All Women Need to Know About Body Positivity." *Woman's Day,* January 27, 2017. http://www.womansday.com/health-fitness/advice/a57752/what-is-the-body-positive-movement, accessed July 31, 2017.

*Bettie Page Reveals All.* Directed by Mark Mori. 2013. Chicago, IL: Music Box Films, 2013. DVD/Blu-ray.


CHAPTER FOUR:
**THE BODY**

Sharkey, Lorelei. "Not the Pin-Up We Played Her For: An Interview with Bettie Page." Nerve.com, 1998. http://www.nerve.com/dispatches/page/pinuplegend, accessed July 31, 2017.

Carney DR, Cuddy AJ, Yap AJ. "Power Posing: brief nonverbal displays affect neuroendocrine levels and risk tolerance." *Psychological Science.* October 2010; 21(10):1363-8.

Scarpa S, Nart A, Gobbi E, Carraro A. "Does Women's Attitudinal State Body Image Improve After One Session of Posture Correction Exercises?" *Social Behavior and Personality*. 2011; 39:1045-52.

Rodriguez, Tori. "8 Ways to Keep Your Workouts Body-Positive." Refinery29, May 20, 2016. http://www.refinery29.com/2016/05/111307/body-positive-fitness-tips-motivation, accessed July 31, 2017.

National Institutes of Health. "Benefits of Physical Activity." June 2016. https://www.nhlbi.nih.gov/health/health-topics/topics/phys/benefits, accessed July 31, 2017.

Weir, Kirsten. "The Exercise Effect." American Psychological Association, December 2011. http://www.apa.org/monitor/2011/12/exercise.aspx, accessed July 31, 2017.

Harvard Health Letter. "Exercise Is an All-Natural Treatment to Fight Depression." Harvard Health Publications, August 2013. https://www.health.harvard.edu/mind-and-mood/exercise-is-an-all-natural-treatment-to-fight-depression, accessed July 31, 2017.

CHAPTER FIVE:
**THE BEAUTY, Part I: Vintage Hair & Makeup**

Sharkey, Lorelei. "Not the Pin-Up We Played Her For: An Interview with Bettie Page." Nerve.com, 1998. http://www.nerve.com/dispatches/page/pinuplegend, accessed July 31, 2017.

Adamas, Aneles. "Pinup Beauty: Victory Roll for Medium-to-Long Hair." *YouBeauty*, May 14, 2004. http://www.youbeauty.com/beauty/victory-roll-pinup-hair, accessed July 31, 2017.

CHAPTER SIX:
**THE BEAUTY, Part II: Pinup Style**

"Bettie Page Talks God, Love and Bondage." *American Suburb X,* June 10, 2015 (transcribed from September 1998 interview). http://www.americansuburbx.com/2015/06/interview-interview-with-bettie-page-1998.html, accessed July 31, 2017

Crandell, Ben. "The Real Bettie Page Reveals Herself in New Documentary." SouthFlorida.com, November 27, 2013. http://www.southflorida.com/events/go-guide-blog/sf-betty-page-reveals-all-in-new-documentary-20131127-story.html, accessed July 31, 2017.

*Bettie Page Reveals All.* Directed by Mark Mori. 2013. Chicago, IL: Music Box Films, 2013. DVD/Blu-ray


CHAPTER SEVEN:
**THE BRAINS**

"Bettie Page Visits the Mr. Showbiz Celebrity Lounge." *Mr. Showbiz Celebrity Lounge,* March 1996. http://www.grrl.com/chat.html, accessed July 31, 2017.

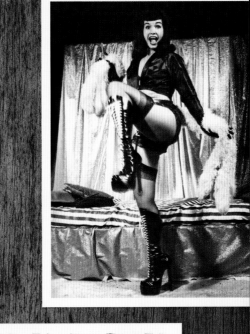
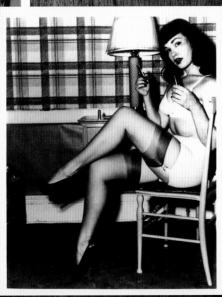

# PHOTO CREDITS

Unless otherwise noted, all Bettie photos shown throughout the book are courtesy of CMG Worldwide. Bettie Page™ is a trademark of Bettie Page LLC (www.bettiepage.com).

### CHAPTER ONE:
### THE BETTIE BABES

Dita glamour, with boa: Shannon Brooke

Dita standing, black lingerie: Shannon Brooke

Madonna: Dimitrios Kambouris / Staff; Getty Images Entertainment

Katy Perry: s_bukley / Shutterstock.com

Angelique Noire: Romain Court

Sunny Moon: Vlad Voloshin

Miss Lady Lace: Luke Wilson Photography

BrittanyJean: Robert Alvarado

Jenny Mostly: Hellcat A-Go-Go Studios

Therése Rosier: Benn Murhaaya

Miss Rockwell DeVil: Susana Clark

Lily Monroe: Frank Lam Photography

Marie Devilreux: Anna Swiczeniuk; courtesy of Bettie Page Lingerie (shown on model) by Playful Promises

Madeline Sinclaire: Janet Barnett

Cheetah Lyn: JJS Photography

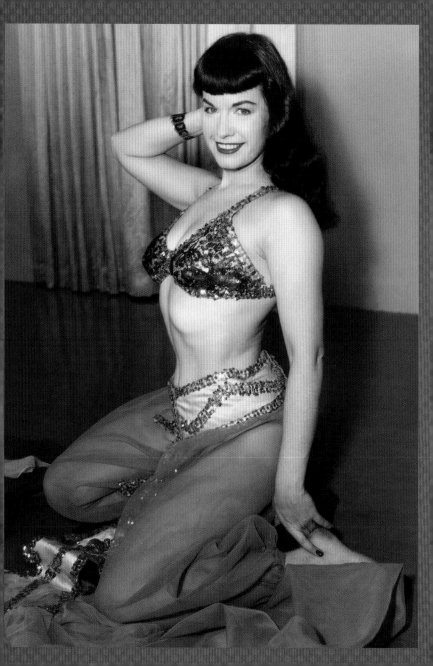

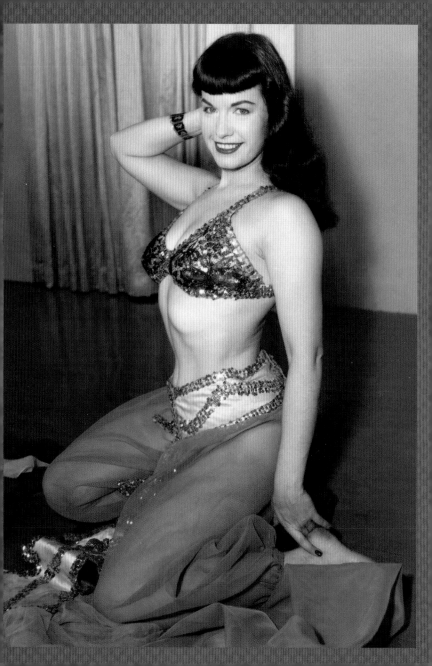

CHAPTER TWO:
**THE BACKSTORY**

Bettie's yearbook photo, Bettie and Goldie, and the two pre-bangs
 Bettie photos: courtesy Mark Mori, *Bettie Page Reveals All*


CHAPTER THREE:
**THE BOLDNESS**

Angelica Luna: Summer Shea Photography

Ursula Undress: B. Magerko

Lyla Blush: Brooklyn Brat Images

The Diamant Duchess: Brooklyn Brat Images

Vintage Vandalizm: Daniel Rodriguez

Ashleeta Beauchamp: Lars Morris

Evelyn Holloway: Daring Dames Photography

Miss Emmy de la Mer: Jason Holmes of Retrodolls

Whittney Chaplin: Andrew Kepinski


CHAPTER FOUR:
**THE BODY**

Tori Rodriguez: Pearl Davies


CHAPTER FIVE:
**THE BEAUTY, PART I: VINTAGE HAIR & MAKEUP**

Meghi Misfit: Mikey Martinez

Pixie Pineapple: Lyla Blush

Jessica Batiste: Jessica Batiste

Miss Lady Lace: Luke Wilson Photography

The Diamant Duchess: Billy Hawkins

Vanessa Pina: Lyla Blush

## CHAPTER SIX:
## THE BEAUTY, PART II: PINUP STYLE

10 Style Lessons from Bettie Page: Brittany Sherman

Cora Harrington: Anna Swiczeniuk; courtesy of Bettie Page Lingerie by Playful Promises

Stefanie Jones: Brooklyn Brat Images

Brittany Sherman: PJ Sherman

Miss Velvet Wren: Amber Rhodes-Lapoint

Bettie Page Clothing by Coral & Jade: courtesy of Coral & Jade Apparel

## CHAPTER SEVEN:
## THE BRAINS

Photos for all three projects: Brittany Sherman of Vavoom Vintage

Bettie Page painting: Therése Rosier

Miss Taylor Nicole: Red Velvet Photography

Bettie Page Clothing by Coral & Jade: courtesy of Coral & Jade Apparel

Bettie Page Reveals All cover: courtesy of Mark Mori

Kalani Kokonuts and Millie Michelle for Bettie Page Rum and Bettie Page Wines: Radiant Inc

Bettie Page Shoes: courtesy of Bettie Page Shoes by Ellie

Lilla Rosten wearing Bettie Page Bridal: Tara O. Photos

Bettie Page Handbags by Lola Ramona: courtesy of Lola Ramona

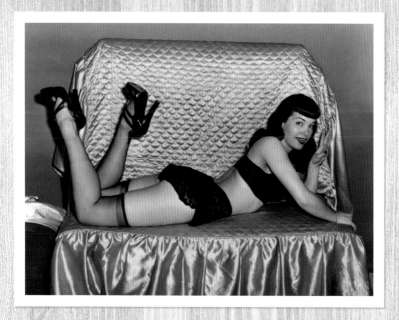

# ACKNOWLEDGMENTS

Many thanks to our beloved Bettie and all who have allowed me the great honor of telling her story and spreading the joy she inspires: El Uno, Mark Mori, Mark Roesler and Bill Uglow of CMG Worldwide, Ron Brem and Goldie Page, Coleen O'Shea, Cindy De La Hoz, Susan Van Horn, and all the Bettie Babes. And, of course, endless thanks to Mom, Dad, family, and friends. Much love to all!

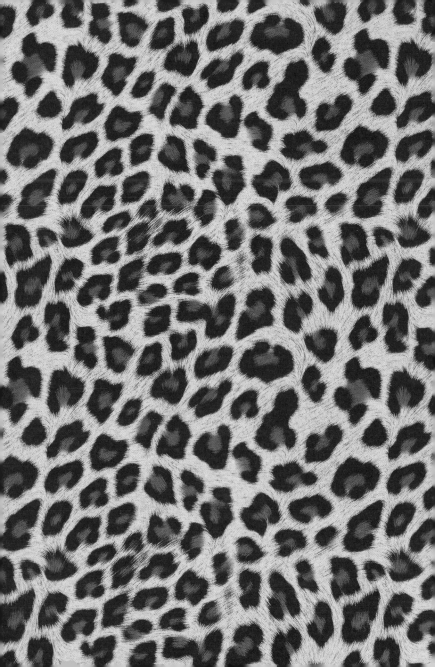